Springer Series on
LIFE STYLES AND ISSUES IN AGING

Series Editor: Bernard D. Starr, PhD
Marymount Manhattan College
New York, NY

Advisory Board: Robert C. Atchley, PhD; M. Powell Lawton, PhD; Marjorie Cantor, PhD (Hon); Harvey L. Sterns, PhD

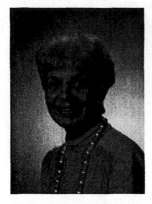

Virginia Burlingame, MSW, PhD, earned her master's degree from Boston University and a doctorate in counseling/psychology from Northwestern University; her dissertation was on the History of the Family Therapy Movement in the United States. She worked in many areas of social work for over 40 years, is a Board Certified Diplomate, and was given Boston University's 'Outstanding Career in Social Work Award' in 1996. She retired from the private practice of clinical social work in marriage, family, and gerocounseling in 1997. She was a clinical member of the American Association of Marriage and Family Therapy.

Dr. Burlingame received a Certificate in Gerontology from the University of Wisconsin-Oshkosh in 1990. As a 1991 Fellow with the Midwestern Geriatric Education Center at Marquette University, her project led to the creation of the Wisconsin Gerontology Institute at UW-Parkside in Kenosha, Wisconsin, and her 1995 minifellowship in ethnogeriatrics at Stanford Geriatric Education Center led to the research and writing of this book. In 1995, Dr. Burlingame interned at Hanley-Hazelden of St. Mary's in West Palm Beach, Florida in their aging and addictions program, and she taught gerontology there in 1996.

As co-director of UW-Parkside's Gerontology Institute, Dr. Burlingame teaches gerontology classes and assists with the Adventures in Life Long Learning and Elder Hostel programs. She writes a newspaper column on Artful Aging.

Ethnogerocounseling

Counseling Ethnic Elders
and Their Families

Virginia S. Burlingame, MSW, PhD

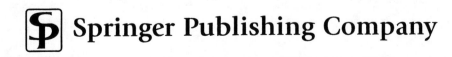 Springer Publishing Company

Springer Publishing Company, Inc.
536 Broadway
New York, NY 10012-3955

Cover design by Janet Joachim
Acquisitions Editor: Helvi Gold
Production Editor: Jeanne Libby

00 01 02 / 4 3 2

Library of Congress Cataloging-in-Publication Data

Burlingame, Virginia S.
    Ethnogerocounseling : counseling ethnic elders and their families
/ by Virginia S. Burlingame.
        p.   cm. — (Springer series on life styles and issues in
aging)
    Includes bibliographical references (p.   ) and index.
    ISBN 0-8261-1217-X
    1. Minority aged—Counseling of—United States. 2. Minority aged—
Family relationships—United States. I. Title. II. Series.
HV1461.B875   1998
362.6'089'00973—dc21   98-28250
                                                                        CIP

Printed in the United States of America

Contents

Foreword

As we look forward to working with older Americans in the 21st century, the reality of ethnic diversity is unavoidable. Projections that one in four of us aged 65 and over in the United States will be from one of the ethnic minority categories by 2030, and one in three by 2050, make it imperative that the predominantly Anglo models of senior services be replaced by multicultural models. Of course, the predictions based on the current prevailing method of counting diversity—assigning individuals to one of the four racial or ethnic minority categories recognized by the census—we know greatly underestimates both present and future ethnic diversity. Among the older adults assigned to each of the four ethnic minority categories used by federal data sources, as well as those in the majority white category, are vast ranges of cultural diversity. This reality makes the work of this volume important and relevant.

From the perspective of providers of mental health services, this complexity is magnified many times over by a few other characteristics inherent to the counseling field:

- not only is the ethnic and cultural diversity of older American clients increasing rapidly, but the diversity of counselors is likewise multiplying, producing countless possible cultural combinations in the counselor-client relationships;
- there are vast ranges of attitudes in the various cultures of the world toward expressing one's feelings;
- there are also vast ranges of attitudes toward revealing one's problems to people who are not members of one's family;
- the current models of counseling used most frequently in the

United States are based on assumptions and principles derived from Northern European or Anglo American experiences, yet the fastest growing cultural groups of older adults are from non-European backgrounds;

- the acculturation level of older clients from cultural backgrounds different from the counselor's is one of the most important attributes in planning a successful approach, but is very difficult to assess before meeting the client;
- and, most importantly, many of the basic processes thought to be critical to the counseling process are almost impossible to accomplish through an interpreter (especially one from the client's family), and yet counselors who speak the languages of the large number of elders who speak little or no English are frequently not available.

For these reasons and many others, this volume by Dr. Burlingame is a most welcome addition to our applied ethnogeriatric literature in mental health. Much of the currently exploding base of knowledge in this area are reports of research recently undertaken as a result of expanded funding by the National Institute of Aging and other public and private organizations. This book represents Dr. Burlingame's effort to translate those findings into useable strategies for counseling older adults. She has also added considerably to the knowledge base by her own interviews with both experienced counselors and older adults from varied ethnic backgrounds.

Particularly valuable insights that readers will find in the following pages are discussions of issues that commonly arise in working with older adults from diverse ethnic backgrounds, and possible methods of addressing them. Some of those issues that I think are most salient are:

- the critical necessity for counselors to know their own cultural background and the biases it likely imposes on their perceptions of their clients' behavior;
- the importance of looking beyond the four ethnic minority categories imposed by methods used by the United States government of collecting and lumping data, to individual cultural groups, in order to find meaningful ways to begin understanding clients' cultural backgrounds;
- the vast array of diverse attitudes and behaviors found within

any one ethnic group, frequently associated with factors such as differences in education, income, religion, geographic region, and acculturation level in the United States;

- the strengths of population groups and the resources they can provide for counselors, as opposed to perceptions of minority groups as those with problems;
- the crucial need to know and understand the historical experience among specific cohorts of elders from different ethnic backgrounds if one is to begin to understand the formative influences they are likely to have had;
- understanding that different cultural perceptions of mental health and goals of relationships, such as harmony and interdependence, may collide with traditional Western assumptions about the goals of therapy; and how those perceptions and goals may help the counselors themselves grow and expand their own sense of values;
- and, the intertwining of spirituality or religion and healing in many of the world's cultures.

This book can be useful in many different contexts and settings, but one of the most obvious is for educational purposes. Two particular attributes enhance its teaching value: 1) the fascinating case histories the author has collected and integrated into the discussion of issues for each of the ethnic categories; and 2) the very specific skills that are recommended for addressing important issues. These skills are clearly based on Dr. Burlingame's own considerable experience as a counselor and her interviews with numerous experienced counselors from various ethnic backgrounds who have worked with older adults.

In short, I am grateful that our delightful and charming former fellow in the Stanford Geriatric Education Center Minifellowship in Ethnogeriatrics, Dr. Virginia Burlingame, has made this major and important contribution to the field in which we work. I am also pleased to recommend this volume to you as a valuable resource to understanding and practicing culturally competent ethnogeriatric mental health care.

Gwen Yeo, PhD, Director
Stanford Geriatric Education Center
August, 1998

Prologue

When I wrote *Gerocounseling: Counseling Elders and Their Families* (1995), I used a Gero Chi Model with case studies from various fields in the health and social service professions; I also tried to incorporate different issues and locales so that the book would speak to almost everyone working with all sorts of elders and their families. Most of the examples were composites from real-life cases, but midway through the book, I realized that I didn't have a case of an Asian-American family or a family from the West Coast. So I created a case about a Dr. Woo in Berkeley and sent it off to the Stanford Geriatric Education Center (SGEC) with the question, "Could this really happen there?" Graciously, they forwarded it on to On Lok's Doreen McLeod, who advised me well.

In the midst of that, Dr. Melin McBride proposed that I come to SGEC for a mini-fellowship in ethnogeriatrics. Once I was there, my adviser, Marita Grudzen, suggested that I apply the Gero Chi Model to see how it worked with ethnic elders and their families. That qualitative research later became the subject of this book. I proceeded to go around the country to learn from actual ethnic providers—who were working with ethnic elders and their families—what they thought was important and unique in their work.

When I wrote *Gerocounseling,* I approached the subject somewhat as an expert, having spent the past 40 years doing individual and family counseling and being involved with recent geriatric-gerontology education. However, I approached the present book as a reporter—for the people whom I interviewed are the real "experts" on ethnogerocounseling.

This is a practical book. I have earned MSW and PhD degrees, a graduate Gerontology Certificate, and fellowships in geriatrics and ethnogeriatrics, acquired mostly from academics who did not have much experience in the trenches, so I was full of academic theory. But I longed for more workable "how to" guidelines. The academic rationale was that if you were well schooled in theory, then appropriate behavior would follow. Not always so, I learned. I desperately needed some ABCs, and so did my continuing-education gerontology students who came for help.

I call these students gerocounselors or, when applicable, ethnogerocounselors. They are the people you often meet at meetings of the American Society on Aging (ASA), the folks in the trenches who are engaged in the actual aging service professions. Their credentials range from high school diplomas to PhDs; some have been in the field for eons and others are fledglings. Most are in the health and social service fields, but others are from law, the ministry, the media, etc. Such diversity makes the creation of workshops and courses challenging, but since diversity is what we are all about, the goal is to speak to all levels hoping not to be overly simple to some or over the heads of others.

Gerontology, a multidisciplinary field, has evolved into a sharing of disciplines, and here, as in my previous book, my hope is to share some counseling techniques that may apply to your clients, or patients. By reading some examples of how a trained counselor might work, you will be able to adapt them to your particular situation.

This book will also look at some principles of ethnogerocounseling with the four major ethnic groups, though in your own work you may see only one of them or may see a totally different population. It is hoped that by gaining some awareness of your feelings about ethnicity and learning some things to look for and ask about, you will be able to generalize these principles.

I discovered many things from the ethnic providers I met and the specific workshops I attended. I learned that I had to truly know and feel comfortable with my own ethnic identity before I could know and be comfortable with anyone else's. I had to acknowledge that my own culture—past and present—has its own quaint ideas, mores, and beliefs about health that are okay with me but may appear "strange" to others. As I read and interacted with different people, I learned to put aside the melting-pot theory that I had previously espoused and adopt a more complex, more accepting view of our complementing, contrasting, sometimes conflicting ethnic reality.

My ethnic sources often said that too much emphasis is placed on ethnic problems and deficits and not enough on social causes—or on strengths. My sources wanted providers from the dominant culture to notice the contributions their groups made to that culture. They also noted that little or no attention was paid to the food of each ethnic group as a means not only of physical nourishment but also of spiritual, social, and cultural nourishment. End-of-life issues were also said to be often neglected; one runs the risk of erring at this sensitive time. This book attempts to introduce some of these themes.

The diagrams of the Ethnic Gero Chi, and Gerocounseling Lenses in Chapter 1 are designed to be copied and made into transparencies to demonstrate the necessity of adding The Ethnic Lens to our understanding of aging persons (Gero Chi) and our methods of helping them (Gerocounseling).

There are also exercises at the end of each chapter, to encourage a class, workshop, or an independent reader to think beyond the scope of this book. Stretch your learning beyond its covers. Try to experience each ethnic culture by attending powwows and ethnic festivals and sharing in ethnic foods. Learn more from your ethnic friends and clients. True empathy is getting your feet wet—or, to change the image, standing in someone else's shoes or moccasins.

Acknowledgments

I wish to thank and dedicate this book to the wonderful people at the Stanford Geriatric Education Center in Stanford, CA who generously assisted me through this project, Staff: Gwen Yeo, PhD, Director, Marita Grudzen, MHS, Melen McBride, RN, PhF, Merry Lee Eilers, MA, and Bernadette Serafin; SGEC Faculty: Dolores Gallagher-Thompson, PhD, Julee Richardson, PhD, and Julliette Silva, PhD.

I also wish to give special thanks to my mentors there: Owen Lum, MD, Manuel Yaniz, PhD, Alice Bulos, PhD, and especially Marita Grudzen, MHS. These ethnic-sensitive, well-informed experts on ethno-gerontology and geriatrics wisely counseled and not only steered me to the relevant literature of the day but also shared their valuable insights to make this book possible. I thank them all, the real "experts" of ethno-gerocounseling.

I also wish to thank Mark Marlaire, MA, Co-Director of the Gerontology Institute at UW-Parkside who assisted in this project, Donald Lintner, MA, UW-Parkside Media Services, who did the graphics, and lastly, a special thanks to E. Percil Stanford, PhD, for permission to include his poem, *Awakening,* and to the wonderful people at Springer who helped make this book possible.

PART I

Ethnogerocounseling

AWAKENING

Dreams rush in
Searching, wondering where they end.

Soaring, floating as if a cloud
No pain, no fear, the urge to laugh aloud.

At the moment, no limits known
Now to reap the benefits of seed sown
Good deeds, high hopes intimately grown.

Chased by thoughts of what could be
The struggle within-to stay or flee.

Ah, at last, barriers forced aside
No longer shackled by the mighty tide.
Ready to challenge the world, the unknown, in one great stride.

Awake, awake, ever aware of the distant call
Faint, yet urgent, no time to stall.

Why go? Why seek!?
With certainty it is not for the meek.

Mammoth are the risks to endure
Only to reach the unknown shore.
Walk with pride through the open door.

What is it to know, to share once there
Too often without cause, greeted by a stare
No thought to ask what talents and skills were brought to share.

Awake, awake in a new land
Soar among the clouds, run freely in the sand.

Absorb the new-blend with the old
Tis only the beginning of fortunes untold.

Never too early or late in life to penetrate the unforgiving wall
Awaken, follow those dreams, heed the faint and urgent call.

Adorn the cloak of success
Everyone knows, you've done your very best!

E. Percil Stanford
March 1996

Chapter 1

The Ethnic Lens

This book is about ethnogerocounseling (EGC). *Ethno*, a prefix borrowed from the Greeks, means culture, race, or people. *Gero*, another Greek prefix, means old age. Briefly, counseling is the art of helping people help themselves, so EGC is the art of helping older ethnic people and their families help themselves.

Ethnicity and aging have many commonalties. Both result in significant losses and are notably marked by diversity. Ethnic people, already incredibly diverse, are becoming more so; and there is more variability among older people than any other age group—so each person, family, and culture, must be regarded as unique. Another commonality—and a premise of this book—is that both should be causes for celebration!

While older persons are like other human beings across the life span, we know that there are specific processes and tasks that are unique to aging. The Gero Chi Lens (Figure 1.1) was designed to help us to think about certain relevant aspects of aging. We are wise to tailor our services specifically to fit elders, as the Gerocounseling Lens (Figure 1.2) suggests (Burlingame, 1995). Likewise, despite their commonalities, ethnic groups have specific differences, that affect the aging process and so the Ethnic Lens (Figure 1.3) must be layered onto the Gero Chi and Gerocounseling Lenses if we are to be effective in helping these persons and their families.

Using as examples the four major ethnic groups of the U.S.

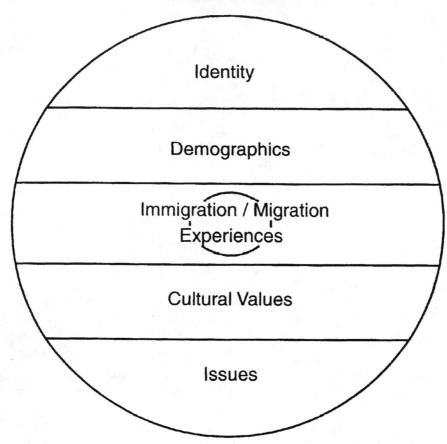

FIGURE 1.1   The Ethnic Lens.

Census—American Indian/Alaska Native (AI/AN), Hispanic-Lati-no (H-L), African American (AA), and Asian/Pacific Islander (A/PI)—this book attempts to highlight some principles of under-standing and providing services to minority elders. Most have been subjected to losses, prejudice, and racism in varying forms and degrees because of experiences resulting from immigration to the United States With linguistic, physical, and cultural traits that make them visible and identifiable, they are underrepre-sented and are often considered "inferior" by others, and "un-worthy" of equal access to power. They therefore are at an increased risk of poor education, poor health, poverty, substand-ard housing, and malnutrition.

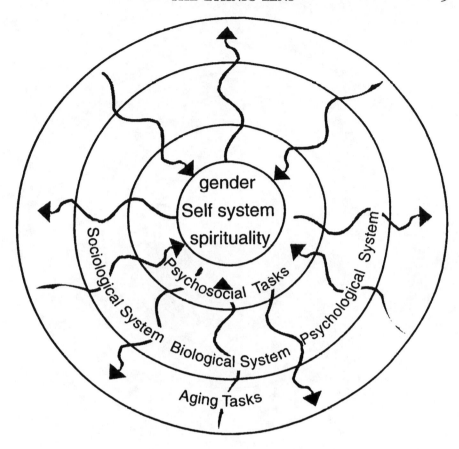

FIGURE 1.2   The Gero Chi* Lens.
*Gero-Circular/Holistic/Interactive

Understanding Ethnicity

The United States has not, as some people suppose, evolved into a melting pot, salad bowl, mosaic, rainbow, or tapestry. We are a diverse, multicultural society, a dynamic mixture of complimentarities, contrasts, and conflicts. The many dimensions that separate us include cultural beliefs and mores, gender, social class, and health—and these differences create both obstacles and opportunities.

Ethnicity, briefly, is an identification with a group that shares common features—language, origin, customs, history, values, and a racial, cultural, or national identity—that differ from those of the dominant culture. It is not a romanticized category of quaint traits

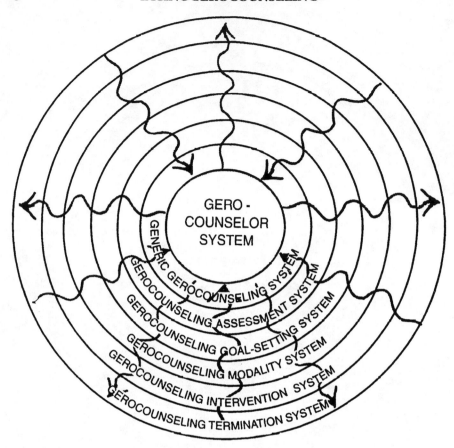

FIGURE 1.3   The Gerocounseling Model.

or even a perspective on misery. Rather, it is a transactional boundary, a process of communicating identity and power between groups (Green, 1995).

Many models have been developed to explain ethnicity. We can think of models as the many lenses of a phoropter, an optical instrument with tinted or corrected lenses used to determine and correct vision errors. Using a new, corrected lens can help us see things in a more realistic way. Lenses or models also help us to make sense of and guide our personal and professional lives. In ethnocounseling, the categorical model is still prevalent but others are also noteworthy: Green's (1995) human service model, Locke's (1992) and Sue and Sue's (1990) cross-cultural models, Barth's

(1969) transactional model, Boyle and Andrew's (1989) cross-cultural nursing model, Ho's (1987) and McGoldrick, Pearce, and Giordano's (1982) family systems models, and Devore and Schlesinger's (1991) ethclass model. Your own personal ethnic lens is also important, for you cannot truly understand another culture unless you have an awareness of your own.

EXERCISE

Your ethnic lens guides your own unique view of the world and contributes to your countertransference. It was created by your

1 Ethnic/cultural ancestry
2 Ethnic/cultural knowledge
3 Ethnic/cultural pride
4 Ethnic/cultural pain

ROUND ROBIN: Split the group and gather in two concentric circles. Each member finds a partner in the other circle. Partners tell each other about their ethnic/cultural backgrounds (5 minutes). Inner circle moves one person to the right.

Repeat.

Move again. Tell your new partner what you know about your ethnicity/culture. Move and repeat. Move right again and tell new partner about your ethnic pride. Move and repeat again (5 minutes each time).

Move once more. Tell each other about racism that you have seen or experienced and how you felt about it. Move one last time and repeat. Discuss or write in your journal what you learned and felt about the exercise. If you are reading independently, imagine yourself in a diverse group experiencing this exercise. What might you have experienced?

The Ethnic Lens

Each ethnic category is in itself a phoropter of ethnic lenses and its lenses help to mold the individuals in the subgroups within it. Since it would be impossible to review all of the ethnic categories in the United States, I hope that the lenses of the four major ethnic categories will yield some general principles regarding cultural sensitivity, which can then be applied to other categories.

Also, since it would be impossible to look at all of the important dimensions of each ethnic lens, five salient dimensions have been used: (1) identity, (2) demographics, (3) immigration-migration experiences, (4) cultural values, and (5) issues. As already noted, the Ethnic Lens will be layered onto the Gero Chi and Gerocounseling Lenses in later chapters.

Identity

The quest for and reaffirmation of identity are played out at times of major life transitions such as adolescence, marriage and divorce, aging, and immigration. This is a dynamic process of interactions with other persons. Identity says where our roots lie, where we've been, who we are now, and what we are becoming in relation to others.

Social identity begins with naming. People wish to be addressed politely by their correct names and titles. But this can be tricky! What people wish to be called depends on their cohort and its circumstances, on present geography, on countries and cultures of origin, on political and economic conditions. Wishes and rules can differ, even within families, because names are not only polite forms of address but also deeper personal expressions of who we are. To avoid offending, if you are in doubt about how to address an ethnic elder, always ask first. When you first greet ethnic elders, use a formal form of address, in keeping with cohort and ethnic preferences.

Then there is the perplexing problem of what to call the various ethnic categories. This is critical because identity with a group becomes part of one's personhood. Ethnic names reflect roots in the past that affect perceptions of events in the present.

The U.S. Census refers to American Indian and Alaska Native, and most people in this vastly diverse category prefer those terms, or the names of their specific tribes. Here, we shall also use AI/AN for brevity. (Native American means anyone born in America.)

Naming blacks depends on the age of the person. Many people aged about 70 years and over still call themselves colored, and some aged 60–69 years prefer Negro—but you would appear prejudiced if you used either term. People aged, say, 59 years and under tend to prefer black, Afro-American, or African—American but again, be careful. People born in Haiti or the Caribbean Islands often prefer names indicating their country of origin (AARP, 1990). Here, we will use black and African American (AA) interchangeably.

Finding a politically correct name for Hispanic-Latino is difficult. Hispanic is often considered a term of the last two decades, Latino the term of the future. AARP (1990) wrote that Hispanic is preferred by Puerto Ricans and Cubans on the East Coast and Latino is preferred on the West Coast, where Chicano is also used by more militant young people. Hispanic is not a racial term; Latino can include Caucasians, American Indians, Africans, and people of mixed ancestry. Some prefer using "country of origin," "heritage," or "Spanish speaking/Spanish surname."

Asian and Pacific Islander is a census term that describes only the geographic base of more than 20 diverse populations. Oriental, coined by the British, is political and is no longer used. Here, we shall use Asian and Pacific islander (A/PI).

Identity is also related to birth cohort, which is more specific than generation. Cohorts contribute to the vast diversity of older persons. It is assumed that people born within a ten year span that encompasses one's coming of age (about age 17–23 in the United States) share the same significant historical events, and therefore share many attitudes, values, and behaviors.

Cohort is often confused with other factors, causing countless myths. A certain work ethic, religiosity, feelings about racism and discrimination, moral and social attitudes, and consumer and financial behaviors are usually time-related cohort affects. If "old age" begins around age 65 and the life span is 125, aging can represent six or more cohorts. The effects of the Depression on your client, for example, were different if he or she was 4 years old, a 14-year-old who had to take a part-time job to help out, or a 20-year-old who had to give up college and postpone marriage, or a 34-year-old who had to keep bread on the table. Is the client's present unwarranted financial insecurity a result of aging or cohort?

Or, similarly, a nursing home resident who rarely was seen naked by a spouse, may feel violated when bathed and taken to the toilet by a black nurse of the opposite sex and may respond with a racial slur that his or her cohort used years ago in emotionally-heightened situations. Richardson (1996) asked if this response is racial prejudice or a cohort effect or both.

Each of the following parts will present a chronological list of major historical events that affected people in each ethnic category. Study them and reflect on how those times and events continue to affect different cohorts. You may find that blacks who lived through the days of Jim Crow and the leadership of Martin Luther King see racism differently from their grandchildren; and women who were suffragists may not always regard political participation as their grandchildren do.

Understanding a people's past, through a lens that includes cohort, is as important as understanding their present. With the American Indian, for example, the total present context is ancient, ritual, political-historical, *and* contemporary.

EXERCISE
Draw a time line of the 20th century. Mark significant economic, political, and social events (Depression, assassinations of King and the Kennedys, wars, sexual and women's revolutions, TV, Elvis, blue jeans, flower children, Reagan years, etc.). Trace on the time line where your grandparents were at various ages. Your parents. Yourself. Interpret cohort affects.

Demographics

Much can be learned about an ethnic group by studying demographics, but a problem in the study of ethnicity and aging has been a lack of research, particularly longitudinal studies, on elders of color. Above all, there are very few data on the AI/AN or A/PI categories. The National Center for Health Statistics which collects mortality data did not even begin publishing those statistics on AI/ANs or A/PIs until 1996, for example. What reports exist elsewhere are often unclear as they tend to lump different ethnic subgroups together.

Another problem is that the 1990 U.S. Census was accused of missing 2.1% of people in the following categories: elderly, minority, ethnic, homeless, undocumented aliens, and poor persons. Thus it is believed to have omitted 5.0% AI/ANs, 5.2% H-Ls, 4.8% AAs, and 3.1% A/PIs, evidently because of linguistic, legal, cul-

TABLE 1.1 Demographic Trends: 65+ Population

Topic	Whites	AI/AN	H-La	AA	A/PI
% Population					
Per Category	14	6	5	8	6
Total US 1990	86.7	0.3	3.7	7.9	1.4
Total US 2030	74.6	0.5	10.9	9.1	5.0
Men per 100 Women	67	73	71	63	82
% Men Married	76.8	60.5	74.9	54.7	82.1
% Women Married	41.8	43.4	36.5	25.5	41
% Residency Non-Metropolitan	27	53	11	21	7
Education					
% High S.	56	34	27	27	47
% None	1	10	10	3.5	10
% Employed	12	11	13	12	16
% Below Poverty Level	10	20	22.5	34	13
Life Expectancy	75.2	71.1	73.3	67	NA

Source: From various reports on U.S. Census.

tural, outreach, and conduct barriers. This is important because policies and programs are then often based on research data about elders in the dominant culture (AARP, 1996).

Age has been called the great equalizer, but the truth is that today's older ethnic population is a very diverse group with significant differences in income, health, and social supports—all affecting quality of life. While statistics reveal many problems and deficits, it is well to know that many ethnic older persons are highly successful by the standards of the dominant culture and their own cultures. Table 1.1 is a composite of data from the 1990 Census.

Immigration-Migration Experiences

Important to the understanding of your ethnogeroclients are their experiences related to immigration and migration. Coming to this country as a new immigrant was drastically different for those who planned, prepared, and saved ahead to join supportive relatives here, compared with others who jumped into a boat to escape death, frightened and feeling alone, not knowing the whereabouts of loved ones. The immigration experience not only reveals some of the traumas with which people have coped but their present strengths and resources.

Immigrants came for varying reasons: economics, employment,

political persecution, natural disasters, criminal prosecutions, etc. Some, such as the Indo-Chinese in the 1980s, were refugees escaping civil strife. Others, such as Mexican agricultural workers, were migrants, crossing borders for employment or to join families.

Timing of immigration was also important in both the host and the home countries. American immigration history is often described in terms of pull and push tactics. Many immigrants were pulled here by the United States' economic needs and other forms of self-interest. When there were labor shortages, as in the building of the transcontinental railroad, gold mining, and seasonal agricultural operations, the United States lured cheap labor from other countries. When employment rose, we conveniently pushed them back home. When the United States saw a small communist neighboring island as a political danger, we welcomed Cubans in with open arms; in the 1990s, when the threat diminished, we became less hospitable.

The history of American immigration practices has been inconsistent. Ironically, despite an immigrant heritage, the evolving dominant society has not always felt warmly about sharing this land with peoples much different from itself. Immigrating colonists treated American Indians already here as inferior outsiders, and Indians and Africans were not even considered whole humans. In the 1930s and again in the 1990s, Mexicans lured here as cheap labor were sent back when they were no longer needed and wanted.

The United States' treatment of Asian immigrants is a case in point. Thousands of Chinese came to the United States during the Gold Rush, but when the need for labor lessened, the Chinese Exclusion Act was passed in 1882, banning new Chinese immigrants and creating (along with anti-miscegenation laws) a Chinese American society consisting of family-deprived bachelors. Many discriminatory laws and practices followed, including the internment of Japanese Americans in World War II (while thousands of loyal Asians were serving in the American armed forces). Such laws were finally repealed in 1943, but the yearly quota for Chinese immigrants was set at only 105. Asian wives were not allowed to immigrate until 1965, when amendments to the Immigration and Nationality Act repealed the original quotas and ended severe restrictions on Asians.

While the goal of the 1965 Immigration Act was the reunification of families, it favored people with American relatives; it also favored skills in elite occupations needed by the Unitd States. Between 1971 and 1980, 75% of new immigrants came from Latin America and Asia. Chinatowns proliferated in San Francisco and New York City; Filipinos migrated to Hawaii and San Francisco's mission district; Koreans settled in Los Angeles and New York City; and the Vietnamese moved to California, Minnesota, and Wisconsin. Major cities became international hubs and the melting pot became a multicultural maze.

In 1986, President Reagan signed a new Immigration Reform and Control Act legalizing certain undocumented aliens who had already established themselves in various ways. In the 1990s, on the coattails of welfare reform, there was a new anti-immigrant movement spearheaded by California's Proposition 187 (1994), which was designed to outlaw illegal aliens and deny them government benefits. At the turn of the new century, prospects for immigrants again look bleak.

Immigration, high fertility, and increased longevity will expand the numbers of ethnic-minority elders in the coming years, with three groups emerging: (1) the native born, (2) people who immigrated when young, and (3) those who arrived as older persons.

Cultural Values

One way to show respect for cultural diversity is to learn about the cultural backgrounds, customs, and values of your minority clients. This requires empathy and a real paradigm shift, as you get out of your own mind-set and into that of another person. You must start by knowing about the dominant culture and your own (if it is different), for we usually define others in relation to ourselves.

Simply, culture is a society's worldview: rhythms, patterns, conduct, values, and skills that are socially acquired through symbols such as customs, techniques, beliefs, institutions, and material objects. Culture is usually transmitted by a language through which members learn, experience, and share their traditions. Culture influences behaviors, social relations, motivation, perception of the world, self, and—yes—the reaction to you and your services.

Each culture has its own way of defining a normal, healthy, psychologically sound individual and family, and its own ideas about how and why an "unhealthy" individual or family should be treated. It sets its own rules for acculturation, defining a commu-

TABLE 1.2   Cultural Values

Dominant Culture	Ethnic Culture
Achievement, success	Harmony
Activity	Passive observation
Competition	Cooperation
Direct	Indirect
Emotional expression	Emotional restraint
Equality, egalitarian	Hierarchy
Family nuclear	Family extended
Future orientation	Past, present orientation
Independence	Interdependence
Individual over group	Family, clan over self
Informality	Formality
Linear	Circular
Nature to be conquered	Nature to be a part of
Personal control	Fate
Optimism	Fatalism
Privacy	Openness
Progress, change	Tradition, stability
Racism; group superiority	Tolerance
Science, rational, secular	Birthright inheritance
Focus on youth	Focus on elders
On time, rigid	In time, fluid

nity, and belonging, as well as rules for family care, child care, and elder care. Various cultures have different attitudes toward age and aging. The rights, obligations, problems, and opportunities of the aged vary across cultures.

Your geroclients will probably be more traditional than their offspring—who are likely to experience more acculturation and intermarriages. Table 2.1 helps us to compare some traditional values of the dominant culture with those of some (though not all) ethnic minorities.

With such a long list of differences, it is no wonder that diverse groups have problems understanding one another—and it is clear why the gerocounselor's task of stepping into the client's shoes is so complex and challenging.

We may be judgmental of other people's customs because we do not understand the underlying values. For example, the dominant culture values personal property and shows this through appearances—well-manicured lawns; neat, orderly front sidewalks. The yards of some American Indian homes may look different: old cars on the grass, disorderly driveways. Do "they," as some people think, not care or do they care about different things? Instead of acquisitiveness for personal property and appearances, do they show caring through reverence for and preservation of the larger environment—nature? Are most of them polluters (like so many in the dominant culture)? Are old cars and similar items lying around indications of poverty and overcrowded housing with no garages and little storage space?

When your Hispanic-Latino client is late for your appointment, is it because she does not value your service or because she puts more value on people who need her, particularly her family? Is she late because she stopped to listen to a troubled family member?

To do a good job with a very different culture, you need to see that "their strange, weird ways; quaint, cute customs; or irrational or inconsistent beliefs and practices," as commonly stereotyped, were probably based on very sound reasons and beliefs. In self-discovery, you may also find that your own culture too has some ways, customs, beliefs, and practices that may appear "strange, weird, quaint, cute, irrational, or inconsistent" to an outsider.

EXERCISE
Record in your journal some of the traditional spiritual, dietary, health, and healing practices that your family or group have that may seem out of the mainstream. What are some of your myths? What do you do for good luck? How do you rationalize? What do you fantasize about? What tricks and techniques are used for coping?

Issues: Sources of Pride and Pain

Many people who write about ethnicity and aging contrast the demographics of ethnic elders with those of whites and focus on problems and deficits. These writers neglect accounts of the richness of ethnic cultures, their secure sense of belonging to a cohesive group, their pride in being linked to an ancient history, the pleasures derived from cultural symbols, and the benefits of being "ethnic." Instead, ethnic elders are often portrayed as recipients of services, disadvantaged and needy; and ethnicity is seen as the cause of a group's problems rather than as one of the solutions.

The truth is that because of their ethnicity, immigrants were forced to develop strength in order to survive, and their ethnicity also served as a buffer against stress and even against the problems of aging.

"Diminished identity" is often experienced in aging as a result of multiple role losses; but it appears less often among ethnic groups that recognize an ongoing need for their elders to actively participate in family roles such as grandparent. In the dominant white society, roles are linked to chronology; in ethnic societies, they are often linked to competence and need.

Ethnicity requires elders to be flexible and adaptive, to utilize whatever resources they have, and to develop new resources in order to survive in an often heartless world. The extended family, fictive kin, and religious and social organizations function as resilient networks in which elders do not have to become isolated or obsolescent because their skills are outdated.

Having survived, ethnic elders bring wisdom, cultural diversity, experience, and productive capacities to aging and serve as important resources in their groups. They function as keepers of tradition, as role models, as sources of cultural cohesion, as teachers, caregivers, mediators, superegos, and facilitators.

Ironically ethnicity is often blamed for keeping immigrants in service work areas, but those very same positions prepare ethnic elders for a retirement wherein service to others continues as a way of life. This is often in contrast to the dominant culture's concept of retirement as the end of responsibilities.

Ethnicity, always emerging, provides a future to others; aging may mean adaptation to dark inevitability. Ethnicity calls not for adaptation but for "surviving, continuing the good struggle, overcoming"—and these words are often heard.

Ethnicity lends pride and the "underdog's pleasure" one feels when fellow group members, despite the odds, reach the top, or simply when they are visible serving their new country in the government or the armed forces.

It is unfortunate that when problems among ethnic peoples are listed, causes such as racism, adverse economics, broken promises, and unmet expectations are seldom reported. And when even their strengths are acknowledged, these strengths have sometimes been used *against* ethnic groups—we hear falsehoods such as, "They don't need help; they prefer taking care of their own," or, "They are a model minority; they have no problems."

There are many indicators of pain as well as pride among ethnic groups that warrant recognition. Higher rates of poverty, poorer health and lower rates of health, shorter life expectancies, substandard housing, inadequate transportation, less education, and less facility in English are seen. This ethnic pain as well as the pride will be discussed in subsequent sections.

EXERCISE

1 What are the official identities and titles of your ethnic groups? What do these names mean?
2 How have the demographics of your ethnic groups affected you or your family?
3 What were your ancestors' experiences in their home countries?
   What did you or your ancestors experience in the host country?
4 List some basic values of your ethnic groups. What stereotypes and myths exist about them? What special problems, issues, pain prevail? What specific resources, strengths, and contributions emerge from your ethnic groups?

Chapter 2

The Gero Chi Lens

Today, individuals of all ages are viewed as biopsychosocial beings, but the Gero Chi Lens (see Figure 1.1)—a circular, holistic, interactive lens—helps us to understand aging persons even more specifically. A systemic approach to viewing elders, it emphasizes the fact that while there is great variability in this population, there are certain observable distinctions and similarities regarding cohort and aging.

Each system within the geroclient system is important, of course; and each, being systemic, interacts with the others in a circular (nonlinear) way. It is impossible to describe this adequately in a brief overview of aging—the subject would take volumes—but that is not the purpose of this book. The discussions of aging systems in this chapter and subsequent chapters are meant to be only brief summaries.

A second purpose of this book, as already noted, is to add the Ethnic Lens onto the Gero Chi Model, to see what changes must be made in our perceptions and in our work with ethnic elders. The pages ahead will tell a part of that story; but again, remember we are seeing only a part of a much broader picture. It is hoped that noting a few unique aspects will enhance your awareness and spur you on to seek more.

The Self-System

The self—a rich, complex process—is a unique composite expression of all that one is and all that one is becoming or has the potential to become. It is important in aging, a time when a changing self-concept can often affect self-esteem. Two additional facets of the self are also noteworthy here: gender and spirituality. All of these concepts are systemic, as they affect and are affected by each other and by all other systems.

The individual, independent self is at the center of the dominant culture's model, but when we apply the Ethnic Lens to the Gero Chi, alterations begin immediately. For American Indian/Alaska Native Americans (AI/AN), instead of self, the basic unit becomes the family-clan-tribe; for the Hispanic-Latino Americans (H-L), it is the self within the family. The African American (AA) self is an interdependent self in a flexible family system; the Asian/Pacific Island American (A/PI) self changes to diminished self in extended family.

Self-concept, the cognitive definition of one's identity, is usually based on life roles and expectations about oneself and others; and in all four of the major ethnic categories, such role responsibilities are clear. The interdependent AI/AN self shares importance with all aspects of nature; the H-L, while placing high value on *personalismo,* stresses *familismo.* The AA self has been described as struggling to maintain a bicultural balance between two antithetic worlds, and the affiliative Asian American self has responsibilities to a structural order that even includes ancestors.

Self-esteem, the emotional evaluation of oneself, is both injured and enhanced in an ethnic person. While a revived emphasis on ethnic solidarity and pride promotes esteem, racism from the dominant society demotes it and puts it at risk.

Gender

Aging is experienced differently by men and women. Gender is tied closely to self-concept and self-esteem, and it helps to determine "who I will become." Despite recent societal modifications of prescribed gender roles in the dominant culture, one's gender still holds a significant place in our lives, including the lives of elders and especially the lives of ethnic older persons. Additionally, many older women in our ethnic categories did not experience what has been called "women's liberation," and they therefore bring their unique cultural gender issues to aging.

Most older women of all categories, including whites, are more likely than men to be single, isolated, lonely, and deprived of caregivers, and to feel that they are no longer valued sexually. Because of early discrimination in various areas, many approach aging with limited resources such as pensions and insurance; and because they live longer than men, they are subject to more chronic illnesses (usually not covered by insurance). However, most show strength through ongoing relationship and social skills.

Older men, who on average die seven years earlier of more acute causes (but with more insurance coverage for hospitalization, and caregivers), have alarmingly high rates of depression and suicide. These have been attributed to incongruities between the older male's ideal self and the losses of advancing age. Other factors, such as retirement and widowhood, when linked to a lack of self-care, social and relationship skills, leave many older males, white and ethnic, unprepared for aging.

Spirituality

If gender provides energy to the self, spirituality provides organization—it is a process by which one organizes all that one is. And just as gender encompasses more than sexuality, spirituality includes more than religion. *Spirituality,* here, refers to how one views life and all of its meanings. Older persons, like others, experience spirituality in a variety of ways; and as spiritual and religious views are often a foundation for coping, relating, and handling suffering and death, they are most relevant to gerocounseling.

Many ethnic spiritual systems are hybrids that combine spiritual beliefs and traditions of ancient cultures with today's modern habits, such as church-related customs. For example, the spiritualism in black churches, Christian or Moslem, with their strong African antecedents, is often cited as continuing resources that meet the biopsychosocial as well as the religious needs of their members. In Asian societies, Confucian, Hindu, Buddhist, and Taoist philosophies permeate not only Christian (and other) religions but also

everyday practices. Most American Indians synthesize their spirituality to include worship in churches of the dominant society along
with the beliefs and traditions of ancient Indian times. While most
Hispanic-Latinos are Roman Catholic, H-L spiritual beliefs remain
influenced by Spanish, African, and American Indian belief systems.

The spirituality seen in most ethnic groups is often tied to
beliefs about the causation and healing of disease, about health,
and about other problems. This of course, relates to how your
services will be regarded and received. Knowledge of your clients'
religious and spiritual beliefs will help you to make effective interventions, to draw on strengths and appropriate resources, and to
ensure against offending.

As discussed in Chapter 1, many ethnic elders hang on to old,
traditional healing practices that often fall under the heading "folk
medicine." If they are new to you, some of these practices may
appear odd. But as has already been pointed out, most of us have
some beliefs and coping strategies that would seem strange to
outsiders. Such ideas can be linked to religion, spirituality, super-
stition, family history or other histories, or even science. Whatever
their sources, they usually are held in high regard and viewed with
reverence, and they should not be dismissed as "cute," "quaint,"
"ignorant" or described by any other demeaning adjectives.

When I asked questions about H-L *curanderos* (see Chapter 7),
for example, most respondents said, "Oh, we don't believe that
anymore," but I discovered that many H-L elders did hold on to
such beliefs. And while I have cognitively rejected some of my
family's early ethnic ideas, they are still a part of my unconscious
and continue to influence me.

Many AI/AN practices, for example, are tied to a respect for
spirits of the dead; some AAs, like Hispanic-Latinas, see spiritual
benefits coming from suffering (this is based on a long history of
physical and emotional pain), and many older H-Ls embrace a
rich, spiritual health belief system regarding health—the *curanderismo* mentioned above. Many A/PI elders continue to use the
Asian medical system based on yin and yang, and other practices
that we call alternative medicine; some combine these with western medicine. No two elders are alike, and no two ethnic elders
are alike; but you will probably observe that your older ethnic
clients are more traditional than their younger relatives.

Psychosocial Tasks

Erikson's (1950) model of psychosocial tasks is often cited in the literature of gerontology to demonstrate that growth and development continue through life. Thus the older person is not only focused on a new Ericksonian task—the balancing of integrity versus despair in order to achieve wisdom—but is also working on unfinished business from earlier stages. The need to feel competent, faithful, loved and loving, and caring (or generative) as well as hopeful, assertive, and purposeful continues through life and perhaps intensifies with the challenges of aging.

Erikson's psychological tasks are yardsticks to measure the development of the self throughout the life span. They are steps by which one learns rules of family and society in order to qualify for adult and, later, elder status. A child's self-concept is created by his or her parents, but as the child's world widens, this self-image, modified by the larger society, is also influenced by one's historical context or cohort experiences—processes that can in turn be influenced by immigration and ethnicity.

The Ethnic Lens makes modifications in this part of the Gero Chi because a particular ethnic culture values each of the psychosocial goals differently, and the unique ways in which these goals are achieved also varies—for instance in childrearing and elder care. To truly understand your ethnic elder clients, it is helpful to learn about traditional child rearing and elder care in their ethnic groups. This will also suggest any conflicts they may be having with children and grandchildren who are adapting to the dominant culture in different ways.

There is little formal research on the application of Erickson's psychosocial model to the four broad ethnic categories; but descriptions of the development of minority-group children (Powell, 1983) and consultations with experts in the field shed light on ethnic clients and their relationships with their offspring. This will be discussed in subsequent chapters. The psychosocial goals and tasks are:

Hope   (trust versus mistrust)
Will   (autonomy versus shame)
Purpose   (initiative versus guilt)
Competence (industry versus inferiority)

Fidelity   (identity versus diffusion)
Love   (intimacy versus isolation)
Care   (generativity versus stagnation)
Wisdom   (integrity versus despair)

The Subset Systems

The Biological System

The term *biological system*, as used here, includes genetics, sex, physical growth and development, treatments and remedies, current functioning in activities of daily living (ADLs), prevention of disease and maintenance of wellness, and history of illness, trauma, and disease.

> Normal aging, the process of senescence, is the increasing vulnerability of an organism processing through life; normal aging also refers to the changes in later life after the reproductive period. It is a multidimensional process. Beyond this, there is no single theory that predicts aging or the rate of aging in individuals. Because there are so many variations within a single individual, it is believed that biological aging is a result of a wide range of processes created by the interaction of physical, mental, and social systems. Effects of genetics, nutrition, medical care, sanitation, stress, support, lifestyles, and social circumstances must all be considered important, giving testimony to how we lived (and live) and how we age (and die). (Burlingame, 1995, p. 51).

As we will see, the Ethnic Lens has a substantial effect on the biological systems of ethnic elders. Lower health status and lower rates of health care are seen. Higher rates of morbidity make it difficult to earn needed supplemental income. There is less utilization of health services, probably owing to less access to care, less adequate insurance coverage, and less access to Medicaid. Many ethnic elders prefer traditional health care that is usually not covered by health insurance and health programs.

Lowered life expectancy among persons of color also exists in the United States. Many never see old age at all, because of infant mortality, lack of preventive health care, lack of medical interventions, poor nutrition, and stress. The American Indian's life expectancy, for example, is 65 years, compared with 73.3 for non-Indians; and a greater percentage of American Indians die from treatable diseases and accidents: there are 59% more deaths from alcoholism and 233% more deaths from pneumonia (U.S. Bureau of the Census, 1991). At age 45, an American Indian experiences limitations in ADLs comparable to a non-Indian age 65. The following chapters will present similar but slightly more positive data about the other ethnic categories.

The Psychological System

Included in the psychological system are cognition, affective characteristics, coping, and personality—including conscious and unconscious effects. The Ethnic Lens poses several interesting psychological questions.

Are ethnic elders' personalities different from those of whites? Here, cultural values shed light, as culture, through the family, is a major sculptor of personality. One's spiritual philosophy also guides personality development (and deviance), as seen, for instance, in various Asian groups. Suicide, for example, is acceptable to Buddhists, and suicide rates are high among the Japanese, Vietnamese, Hmong, and some others.

What defines mental health? Does the definition necessarily include an appropriate adaptation to the dominant culture? To adapt, must one give up core cultural values? When immigrants refuse to do this, are they mentally ill? In the case of American Indians, are alcoholism and suicide to be considered mental, biological, or social problems?

Behavior is usually described as adaptive or maladaptive. If various cultures have time orientations different from that of the dominant culture, which behavior is adaptive? Or is adaptation a matter of perception, location, or choice? The dominant society fears and isolates the mentally ill; many ethnic cultures are tolerant of a wide range of deviant behavior. What, then, is "ill"?

How is mental health or illness to be measured? Western psychologists apply the scientific method, which involves considering cause and effect through the use of linear measurements. Epidemiologists look at clinic admissions. But even the most objective methodologies can have a cultural bias. For example, one study found more violence in American Indian schizophrenics admitted to southwestern hospitals than in comparable non-Indians. Does that mean that Indian schizophrenics are more violent or that the Indian family system is less prepared to deal with violence than a family from another culture?

Gerocounselors have their own ethnic lenses, and countertransference may interfere with psychological assessments. For example, Lum (1993) wrote that in Chinese Americans affective disorders are often underreported, whereas schizophrenia and manic depression may be overdiagnosed. Certain ethnic behaviors are often misunderstood by nonethnic assessors.

You will discover that rates of some mental illnesses are very low among certain ethnic categories. Epidemiological data on dementia for both Asians as a total category and Hispanics, for instance, are negligible. One can make different surmises: such maladies may be less prevalent, may be misdiagnosed, may be less troublesome to the group, may be more shameful and therefore underreported, or may not have been fully counted because mental health services, for one reason or another, were not accessible.

Studying life satisfaction is a popular but less scientific method of assessing the mental health of the elderly. Life satisfaction is reported as high by most white and (especially) black elders in the United States, but it is reported as low by Hispanic-Latino and American Indians (who also report more chronic illness, worry, and financial and family concerns). But again, are these psychological or social problems?

Drug addiction among the elderly is another point in question: Is it is a social, psychological, or genetic problem? Dangerous drug combinations are seen; and in the dominant society, there are usually two categories of alcoholics among the elderly: long-term alcoholics and late-life problem drinkers who use alcohol to cope with the losses of aging. Older drinkers are affected by smaller quantities of alcohol because of slowed metabolic and nervous systems, because of medications they take, and because of other changes related to aging. This is particularly true of Asians, who, in general, do not metabolize American alcohol products very well. While illegal drugs take the lives of countless ethnic young people, they also afflict elders, and rates of alcoholism (and abuse of other drugs) are high for AA, H-L, and AI older persons.

It is important, when evaluating mental health status of a person from a particular category or group, to ask these questions and to apply the group's meaning system in the assessment process along with other criteria. Throughout this book you will be advised to learn about the belief systems of your ethnogeroclients and their groups. These beliefs influence their view of themselves, their afflictions, the world, you, and your services; and they are important criteria for mental health and life satisfaction assessments. Most important, they will reveal the ethnic strengths and resources on which you may draw as partners in your helping team.

The Sociological System

The aging sociological system seems all-encompassing, and we have dealt with many of its aspects. Already included in the Ethnic Lens are references to geographic, economic, and political residence, as well as historical, cultural, ethnic, racial, and social class contexts. When we think of social systems, we also think of relationship systems, which include a broad range of human relations that have special bearing on an older person's physical and psychological functioning and well-being. Scenarios involving families and late-life marriages—particularly with regard to caregiving—may be played out differently among ethnic families, depending on their degree of acculturation and on their expectations. Friends, fictive kin, *compadres*, clans, tribes, and other informal support systems or resources, along with formal supports (used or unused), all help to shape the experience of aging.

Issues such as health and health care, environmental concerns (from the neighborhood to the world and beyond), work and retirement, finances, religion, and death and dying are also important to all elders but may take on special nuances for ethnic older persons. We will take a look at these from the perspectives of the various ethnic categories, to accustom you to viewing these factors through an ethnic lens.

The System of Aging Tasks

Tobin (1988) reminded us that preservation of the self amidst countless losses is the task or the goal of the very old, and Erikson (1950) wrote of the continuing psychosocial tasks and goals that continue to require attention throughout the life span. Finding a balance between a sense of integrity about how one's life has evolved versus despair that it is nearing an end is an important achievement, which is sometimes called the acquisition of wisdom.

These are the existential issues that underlie all the tasks of aging; but there are also more practical tasks that must be accomplished in these years. The practical problems may be the issues that your clients bring to you:

1 Efficient use of medical, social, and emotional supports.
2 Adjustment to declining physical strength and health.
3 Maintenance of satisfactory living arrangements.
4 Coping with retirement and financial changes.
5 Independence and assertive control of life.
6 Assumption of new community responsibilities.
7 Revised relationships.
8 Adjustment to losses of significant others.

Will the Ethnic Lens change the tasks of ethnic elders? No, not entirely. They face the same challenges as elders in the dominant culture. But because of issues noted in the Ethnic Lens, the challenges are more difficult to meet. And there will be a few "ethnic" differences. With many ethnic groups, for instance, the task of "maintaining independence" must be altered and replaced with the value of interdependence. "Assertive control" may be more a family issue than an individual issue.

Added to the list of the tasks of aging should be a harmonious reconciliation of the ethnic culture and the dominant culture, so that ethnic elders can spend their final days in comfort—culturally—and achieve integrity instead of despair. Whether and how much to acculturate or assimilate is, of course, an individual matter.

EXERCISE
Apply the Gero Chi Model to your own aging or that of your parents and grandparents. Now put your Ethnic Lens on top. How does (will) your unique "ethnicity" affect your aging or that of your family members? Comparing your scenarios with those of the dominant culture, what lens effects do you find particularly significant?

Chapter 3

The Gerocounseling Lens

Is the gerocounseling different for ethnic older persons compared with older persons of the dominant culture? Should it be different? After adjusting the Gero Chi Lens to accommodate the Ethnic Lens, how do we tailor our services to fit these heterogeneous categories?

For answers, let us put the Ethnic Lens onto the lens of the Gerocounseling Model (see Figure 1.2). This too is a circular, holistic, interactive approach. It deals with specific principles and techniques of generic counseling as well as the special handling of assessment, goal-setting, choosing modalities and interventions, and handling terminations that will be most appropriate for elder issues.

All other things being equal, it is of course easier and better to do ethnogerocounseling if you are from the same linguistic and ethnic group as your clients. Efforts are being made to recruit and train counselors from specific ethnic categories; but even so, differences in class and acculturation can enter in, making the work more difficult. In any event, until the number of ethnic providers of health and social service is sufficient to meet increasing needs, the major load of ethnogerocounseling will fall on the shoulders of people from the dominant culture or other ethnic groups. Therefore—just as gerocounselors have learned to swap knowledge with providers from other disciplines and various levels of training in their multidisciplinary field—ethnogerocounselors will need to learn all they can from researchers, ethnic workers, and ethnic clients and their families.

Ethno-Generic Gerocounseling

The basics of generic gerocounseling should apply to all cultures. General principles—such as respecting all clients and avoiding arguments, overinvolvement, taking sides, speaking for someone else, rescuing, and breaking silences—are still appropriate. In ethnogerocounseling some rules are especially emphasized, such as the need to learn about the unique circumstances (including the culture) of each individual client and family; to start where the client is; and, when in doubt, to let the ethnogeroclient lead and show you the way. The Ethnic Lens approach also suggests that our skills in ethics, relationships, and communication take on new nuances when we layer the Ethnic Lens over the gerocounseling lens. While it is difficult to translate habitual ways of working, your motivation to be most effective in helping clients help themselves will no doubt prevail.

Ethics Skills

Beneficence, autonomy, and fidelity should be the ethics of all counselors for all clients. These goals interact in a circular way, and each should be maintained unless there is a stronger overriding moral obligation. For instance, beneficence (doing good) for a person who is at great risk may override granting that person autonomy. Sometimes, however, an acceptable compromise can be reached, which incorporates the needs and values of medical-social ethics and those of the ethnic elder's value system. We wish to do good, grant self-determination, and be confidential, faithful, and trustworthy; but the Ethnic Lens presupposes new approaches to these ethical axioms. An old adage fits here: "different strokes for different folks."

What is considered beneficence in the dominant culture may not be "doing good" in an ethnic culture. This issue raises the question, "Who is the client?" Is the client the individual or the family? The dominant society's basic unit is the individual, and its goal is independence. (This is true even in family therapy. The family system is the client, but insurance and most records are based on an individual model, and a common goal is often separation or differentiation of individual family members.) In most traditional ethnic cultures, the family is the basic unit; the family is considered the client; and the goal is harmony and ongoing interdependence.

Often you, the ethnogercounselor, will be granting the *family* autonomy by giving its members information so that *they* can make informed choices about an elder. This can become complicated in our present systems, which still bases such decisions on individual choice.

In matters of advance directives such as living wills, powers of attorney, and informed consent, specific ethnic, acculturation, and intrafamily differences must also be taken into consideration. Disclosing a serious diagnosis or prognosis may have to be handled differently for some ethnic families, and issues of confidentiality often become blurred.

When our ethical principles are viewed through an Ethnic Lens, we must ask not only what is considered ethical in our profession, agency, or governmental unit, but also what is considered right or wrong, appropriate or inappropriate by ethnic elders and their families. And what if family members are divided on ethical issues?

Agency and bureaucratic rules need to be rethought (when possible) in light of their effects on peoples with different viewpoints. By respecting cultural beliefs, and applying our creativity and remaining flexible, we can find ways to modify existing procedures comfortably.

Relationship Skills

Countertransference is a Freudian term describing the totality of feelings experienced by the counselor, attributable to past and present experiences but activated in counseling. Because countertransference influences our actions toward those we are helping and our responses to them, we should be aware of it. The effect is not necessarily negative, but it can include biases, blind spots, and ignorance.

Historical accounts, present-day media, and even our own experiences sometimes lead us to view various ethnic groups or their behaviors negatively. Such impressions—even when intellectually rejected by the most fair and objective people—make an impact on our subconscious and become part of our countertransference. It is better to recognize them and admit that they exist.

Then, make sure you know about your own cultures. For many readers, your subcultures are based on European-American values. Such values may govern your professional expectations and skills, and they may be far different from the values of your ethnic clients. Ask yourself, for example, whether or not you expect to maintain good eye contact and easy verbalization of feelings with people who find these mannerisms alien or even rude. Does your style of elder care put values such as independence and planning first, even when clients have opposite orientations?

The chapters on the different ethnic categories will stress the need to learn and adjust to the courtesies and the relationship rules of each client and family. But a warning! While you learn about the cultural themes of each category, be careful to avoid stereotyping. Just as all elders are different, all ethnic elders are different—especially in their degree and form of assimilation or acculturation.

Cultural knowledge should make us more flexible, not more rigid; and it will tell us only about potential—not necessarily actual—difficulties, sensitive areas, values, and modes of behavior. We must meet the geroclient as a person first, rather than a case study or an ethnic oddity, and we should constantly recheck for feedback from the client.

Transference, the Freudian term describing the totality of feelings expressed by the client, attributable to past and present experiences and activated in counseling—is also something you will need to understand and handle. Many ethnic elders have a long history of ill-treatment and are fearful and suspicious of providers of health and social services, and of bureaucracies. Future chapters will discuss how such distrust can be handled with each category.

Often, negative transference is due to a lack of understanding. Here, "role preparation" helps. Share preliminary information about the roles of client and gerocounselor, about how talking can lead to solutions, and about the general process of your work. Sue and Sue (1990) reported that ethnic clients who received precounseling information had less tendency to terminate, were more satisfied with the process, and perceived more changes in themselves (p. 187). It boils down to knowing what to expect.

Communication Skills

Here again, the rule of thumb is follow the client's lead in both verbal and nonverbal communication. Each culture has its own styles and nuances of communication, and you should know those of your clients so as not to insult or offend them. The following chapters will highlight some communication styles of each category.

The use of interpreters is a much-debated issue. Most experts advocate the use of both ethnic consultants and interpreters when necessary. Lum (1993), however, warned about the limitations of the translator-generated interview. Translators may:

1. Inadvertently change the focus of the conversation
2. Distort because of a lack of professional knowledge
3. Let their attitudes determine what is worth translating
4. Suppress taboo subjects if the translator is a relative or younger

Generally, most experts do not consider family interpreters reliable. The Brookside Hospital in El Cerrito, California, uses the whole hospital staff as volunteer translators. The Federal Government and many states require hospitals to provide interpreters or risk losing Medicaid and Medicare reimbursements but the laws are vague and the reinforcement is difficult. The New York Times (1997) reported that California, Washington, and Illinois had the most comprehensive systems. But many immigrants there and elsewhere do not know their rights in this regard or are hesitant to file complaints. In an attempt to offer a solution, AT&T has a telephone language line which guarantees 24 hour access to interpreters in 140 languages. Critics say it is too costly for most clinics, the quality is spotty, and that the impersonal voice on the speaker phone is disconcerting to older immigrants (Fein, E., 1997, p. 20).

Ethno-Gerocounseling Assessment

As has been stressed, your first goal in assessment should be to understand your own culture and then move on to learn about your geroclient's values, meaning system, and issues of cultural identity or conflict.

A good assessment also includes an understanding of the client's problem and how the client is organized in the Gero Chi Lens as seen though the Ethnic Lens. Included here, for long-term planning, is knowledge about the client's formal and informal support systems and what ethnic and mainstream resources are available in a continuum of care. The client's assessed ADLs (Katz, Ford, Moskowitz, Jackson, & Jaffee, 1963) and IADLs (Duke University, 1978) can then be placed along the continuum of care. This must be reassessed frequently, and interventions should start slowly and low on the continuum. Such is the course for all elders.

Knowing about the client's belief or meaning systems will help you understand the etiology, present circumstances, and future course of the presenting problem and will guide your goals and interventions.

If a client's belief model, for example, is a social one and sees the problem as a result of a traumatic event such as death, the client may feel like a victim. Attributing the loss to bad luck or fate and seeking wise counsel from you, the client will expect you to be nonjudgmental and sympathetic, and may even expect you to "give permission" to abdicate some responsibility for the problem. This should be done, in the interest of preserving the client's dignity; the client's prolonged mourning should be seen not as neurotic or as a complicated bereavement but as a highly respectable conformity to an ethnic tradition of showing deep emotional attachment to the lost person.

Other belief models offer moral explanations, and the problem is seen as punishment for a moral failure or for some violation of culturally prescribed conduct. You may see such explanations as illogical, but can a belief model be illogical? And is it possible to counter such a model? The following case is an example of going along with a belief instead of trying to change it.

Henry at intake presented severe longstanding depressive symptoms. He had seen many psychiatrists, counselors, and spiritual advisors, to little avail. He spent most of the day in bed, admittedly as a form of self-punishment for youthful masturbation, considered a sin in his religion (Catholicism). Psychiatrists told him his early behavior was normal; priests said God forgave him; but Henry's guilt and need for punishment persisted.

Using his beliefs, the counselor said that since she was not God, she did not know if he was a sinner, so she suggested that they proceed as if his belief was correct. She knew his religion had a built-in system to help with such feelings and pointed out that while he had confessed and repented, maybe his penance was insufficient. She listed a few Catholic saints who dedicated their lives to helping others. Maybe, since the sin was so awful in his mind, he needed more penance. She suggested some volunteer activities. That made sense to Henry.

Henry picked up on these suggestions and got out of bed daily. Today several years later, the counselor often sees his name in the newspaper being honored as an active volunteer, and she reads his letters to the editor written on behalf of his good causes.

Ethnogerocounseling Goals

In all gerocounseling, start with a clear statement of the presenting problem from the client, the family, and the referring person. This is especially true for older ethnic clients, who often present problems in the form of physical or vocational complaints. Sometimes the focus will be on external conditions such as housing, food stamps, or medical care rather than in-depth personal matters; and the processes, goals, and expectations of the white, middle-class gerocounselor may have to be altered to meet the client's expectations. As you agree on an immediate, specific goal, be sure to word it positively, in process form, in the present tense, and in the client's own language so that everyone understands.

But while counselors should initially respond to any seemingly surface but immediate problems in order to establish hard-earned trust in the relationship, you will find that powerlessness is the greatest stressor for most minority people, and therefore empowerment should be a high-priority goal whether it is verbalized or not.

Ethnogerocounseling Modalities

Various counseling modalities have been used with minority older persons, some with more success than others. Because of the importance of the ethnic, interdependent, extended family, family counseling is often considered the "treatment of choice," but owing to practical logistics (work, transportation schedules, etc.), much individual counseling is done. What is important here—in any modality—is outreach.

In conjunction with the goal of empowerment, you will often find yourself in the role of advocate as you access ready resources, work on trying to change the existing system, or refer to appropriate organizations or persons within your elder client's ethnic group that function in this regard. Whether or not you call yourself a case manager, that is what you will often become.

Ethnogerocounseling Interventions

Good gerocounseling interventions incorporate environmental press, parsimony, values, learning styles, gentleness, a systems outlook, use of time, and the old cliché, "Different strokes for different folks" (Burlingame, 1995, pp. 147–155).

Briefly, *environmental press* means that persons perform at maximum levels of competence when environmental pressures (demands of daily life) slightly exceed the level at which they adapt (their competence). *Parsimony* reminds us that the least intervention is the best intervention. A *values* principle (the subject of this book) says that interventions should be chosen within the framework of the client's value system and what the client deems appropriate or inappropriate, right or wrong.

You will also want to tailor your interventions to the client's *learning style* and, of course, practice *gentleness*—that is, refrain from direct, harsh confrontations and indiscriminate disarming. A *systems outlook* will help both the ethnic geroclient and yourself—for when multiple problems appear overwhelming, it is helpful to remember that you don't have to fix everything, that even a small change in one part of the system can lead to changes in other parts.

The *use of time* can itself be converted into an intervention. Despite the recent "managed care" emphasis on brief counseling, most of your clients will fall under the heading of long-term care because their problems will be chronic and possibly progressive. However, brief and long-term counseling do not have to be incompatible. Many gero–case managers and other gerocounselors today function much like traditional family doctors, seeing clients from crisis to crisis and from transition to transition, and being available as ongoing resources—almost like one of the family. Instead of an emphasis on pathology, strengths and resources are evoked to work on the immediate problem. Such solution-focused work usually entails a rapid response and intervention; a clear, shared definition of responsibilities; creative and flexible use of time; and interdisciplinary cooperation with multiple formats and modalities, using referrals for existing services to prevent duplication.

In choosing modalities and interventions with minority elders, Falicov (1982) suggested that you first determine if the problem is cultural, situational, a dysfunctional pattern of cultural transition, or a transcultural dysfunctional pattern.

Cultural patterns look like problems, but they are really part of a culture (belief system, developmental norms, family roles and rules). *Situational* patterns of stress (isolation, lack of information) are at the interface between the geroclient and the dominant society, and here you play matchmaker with community resources to alleviate environmental stress. Along with formal support systems, you may engage extended family and fictive kin and act as an intermediary, educating and empowering the clients but not getting into psychological issues.

Dysfunctional patterns of cultural transition are patterns that were necessary during immigration but have now become rigidified, interfering with adjustment to the dominant culture. An example could be newly-immigrated grandparents—overly strict and protective of their grandchildren because of the dangers in a new country—who are having difficulty relinquishing some control as the children become more acculturated. Conflict results as the children want to become more American too fast and the elders want them to hold on to the old ways too long. Here, you might become a cultural family mediator challenging this dysfunctional pattern as a deviation of their cultural heritage and a barrier to succeeding in the new society. The children who are blatantly disobeying the caregiver grandparents may be warned, "Children do not have as much power in Mexico; you should go back to your old ways" and conversely, the grandparents maybe advised, "Children here have more freedom so you may have to give in a little."

Transcultural dysfunctional patterns are universal problems aggravated by cultural change. For example, when the expected form of care for frail grandparents may become impossible because the extended family no longer exists and all possible caregivers must be in the workforce.

You will find countless ways to introduce ethnic sensitivity and competence into your interventions; this begins with applying the Ethnic Lens to your clients' Gero Chi Model and using the new version to modify your gerocounseling. Just asking a simple, polite question about the client's mores is an intervention—it validates the person and his or her culture and shows your desire to understand and be of help. The next sections will spell out some ways this can be achieved with our four ethnic categories.

Ethnogerocounseling Terminations

As with all older clients, work with ethnic elders will include terminating interviews, closing cases, and also saying good-bye to relationships when clients move to different levels of care or when they die. While there are many differences between and within cultures regarding norms for expressing grief, the experience of loss is universal and you and your clients are no exception. The preliminary information about the counseling process should include your rationale for all termination policies, and this could help to pave the way. Ethnogeroclients and families, unfamiliar with counseling, may see you more as a friend than a professional, and it is important that their expectations are realistic from the start so that they do not feel let down when you terminate.

We have stressed that certain issues may require special handling with ethnic elders, and there is probably no area more sensitive—for individuals and groups—than death and dying. But individuals and cultures grieve in their own unique ways, and therefore our understanding, assistance, and comfort must also be uniquely culture-specific.

It is well to remember that while termination means ending, we never really say good-bye. Your contributions to the future well-being of your ethnogeroclients and the gifts they have shared with you, in terms of learning and cultural enrichment, will stay with you both forever and a day.

Ethnogerocounseling is not easy work. It is hard enough to work with the multiple problems of the aged and their accompanying emotional losses in a present-day chaotic health system, but harder still when we must add an Ethnic Lens, must translate our knowledge to accommodate a new worldview and sometimes another language, and must modify our comfortable work habits accordingly. But the rewards are many. You will be intellectually challenged, in step with the multiethnic 21st century, professionally enhanced, broader, and more sophisticated (in the best sense) if you take this route. There is much to learn from elders, and there is even more to learn from ethnic elders. And most of all, you will have the good feeling of doing the best job you can on behalf of your clients.

References for Part I

American Association of Retired Persons. (1990). *Celebrating diversity: A learning tool for working with people of different cultures*. Washington, DC: Author.

American Association of Retired Persons. (1995). *A portrait of older minorities*. Washington, DC: Author.

American Association of Retired Persons. (1996). *Appreciating diversity: A tool for building bridges*. Washington, DC: Author.

American Society on Aging. (1992). *Serving elders of color: Challenges to providers and the aging network*. San Francisco: ASA.

Barth, F. (1969). *Ethnic groups and boundaries*. Boston: Little, Brown.

Boyle, J., & Andrews, M. (1989). *Transcultural concepts in nursing care*. Glenview, IL: Scott Foresman.

Burlingame, V. (1995). *Gerocounseling: Counseling elders and their families*. New York: Springer.

Devore, W., & Schlesinger, E. (1996). *Ethnic-sensitive social work practice* (4th ed.). Boston: Allyn and Bacon.

Duke University Center for the Study of Aging and Human Development. (1978). *Multidimensional functional assessment: The OARS methodology*. Durham, NC: Duke University.

Erikson, E. (1950). *Childhood and society*. New York: Norton.

Falicov, J. (1982). Mexican families. In M. McGoldrick, J. Pearce, and J. Giordano (Eds.), *Ethnicity and family therapy*. New York: Guilford.

Fein, E. (November 23, 1997). Language barriers are hindering health care. *New York Times*, p. 1.

Green, J. (1995). *Cultural awareness in the human services: A multiethnic approach* (2nd ed.). Boston: Allyn and Bacon.

Ho, M. (1987). *Family therapy with ethnic minorities.* Newbury Park, CA: Sage.

Katz, R., Ford, A., Moskowitz, R., Jackson, B., & Jaffee, M. (1963). Studies of illness in the aged. The index of ADL: A standardized measure of biological and psychological function. *Journal of the American Medical Association, 185,* 914–919.

Locke, D. (1992). *Increasing multicultural understanding: A comprehensive model.* Newbury Park, CA: Sage.

Lum, O. (1993). *Chinese American elders.* Presentation: Historical profiles on African-American, Latino, Filipino and Chinese elders. *Working Paper #12.* Palo Alto, CA: Stanford Geriatric Education Center, 43–50.

McGoldrick, M., Pearce, J., & Giordano, J. (Eds.). *Ethnicity and family therapy.* New York: Guilford.

Powell, G. (1983). *The psychosocial development of minority group children.* New York: Brunner/Mazel.

Richardson, J. (1996). The cohort factor-As important as diversity. *Aging Today, 17* (6), 17.

Sue, D. W., & Sue, D. (1990). *Counseling the culturally different: Theory and practice.* New York: Wiley.

Tobin, S. (1988). Preservation of the self in old age. *Social Casework, 69* (9), 550–555.

U.S. Bureau of the Census. (1991, June 12). Census Bureau Releases 1990 Counts on Specific Racial Groups. *U.S. Department of Commerce News.*

Yee, B. (1991). *Variations in aging: Older minorities.* Galveston: Texas Consortium of Geriatric Education Center.

Yeo, G., Young, J. & Gu, N. (1996). *Demographics and health risks of ethnic minority elders: A resource packet for teaching.* Palo Alto, CA: Stanford Geriatric Education Center.

PART II

American Indian/Alaska Native (AI/AN) Elders

Everything on the earth has a purpose, every disease an herb to cure it, and every person a mission. This is the Indian theory of existence.

Mourning Dove Salish (nd)

HISTORICAL CONTEXT

Ice age	Indians arrive from Asia.
1492	Columbus sails for India, lands in North America. Europeans occupy AI/AN homelands.
1742	Generic Indian wars begin.
1787	Indian land purchased; treaties misunderstood, land undervalued, false promises given.
1812	Andrew Jackson relocates Indians west of Mississippi River.
1824	Bureau of Indian Affairs (BIA) in Department of War.
1849	BIA moved to Deptartment of Interior.
1861–65	Civil War.
1863	Emancipation Proclamation.
1868	United States outlaws enslavement of Indians in southwest
1887	Allotment Act gives each AI family 160 acres; size and quality unsuitable for farming. AIs cannot pay taxes; 90 million acres lost and later leased by BIA to white farmers.
1890	US Seventh Cavalry kills 350 unarmed Indians at Wounded Knee, South Dakota, in final Indian war massacre.
1890	Boarding school era begins.
1906	Burke Act gives land and services to "competent" Indians.
1914–18	World War I.
1921	Snyder Act establishes Indian Health Service (IHS).
1924	AI/ANs gain United States citizenship, federal and state services.
1934	Johnson-O'Malley Act gives federal funds to states for AI/AN education, welfare, medical services, agriculture.
1939–45	World War II.
1950	United States government attempts to terminate reservations.
1955	IHS moved to U.S. Public Health Service.
1964–65	Civil rights legislation passed.
1965	Older Americans Act passed.

1975   Indian Self-Determination and Education Act gives Indians self-government.
1980   Reagan era of fiscal cuts.
1981   Indian Council on Aging formed.
1987   U.S. Supreme Court gives tribes autonomy regarding gambling.
1996   Congress cuts $200 million from BIA.

CASE EXAMPLES

Mary Banks, an Urban, Middle Class AI With Medical Problems and Family Conflicts

Mary Banks, age 59, a high school teacher, lives in Fargo, South Dakota. A Lakota Indian, she officially left the Pine Ridge reservation at age 22 but returns often to visit her family. Mrs. Banks sends monthly checks to her poor relatives, worries about their welfare, and is angry about the mistreatment of her people. Her husband, Doug Banks, is a civil engineer of the same tribe. They have two children, Debbie, 19; and Sam, 16. Mrs. Banks is overweight and has hypertension, aggravated by psychological stress, getting too little exercise, and eating too much fast food. She smokes two packs of cigarettes a day.

When the Bankses left the reservation, they were happy to get out. After studying at a boarding high school, a community college, and then the state university, they saw no future for themselves at home and felt ashamed of the poor living conditions and social problems there. But recently, they have experienced a resurgence of ethnic pride and have become dedicated to keeping their tribal culture not only alive but pure. They now believe that Native American ways, particularly among the Lakota are superior to those of the dominant culture. They forbid their children to date non-Lakota friends, and they send the children back to the reservation every summer to absorb the traditional culture.

The Bankse's newfound ethnic pride is not shared by their children, who say they want a normal teenage life. They are angry and rebellious. Mrs. Banks suspects that they are using alcohol and pot. Their grades have dropped this year.

Such problems are affecting the management of Mrs. Banks's

hypertension, and her doctor has warned her that she is at risk of a stroke if she doesn't reduce her stress and quit smoking. But she says that she cannot do either. She is addicted to tobacco, and she obsesses over the children. The more upset she gets, the more she yells; and then the children act out more, and she worries more, and her blood pressure rises. Her physician has finally referred her to Miriam Wells, a white MSW. Ms. Wells is wondering where to begin.

Margaret Mayflower, a Reservation AI With Depression and Moderate Family Support

Margaret Mayflower, age 80, has lived on a Navajo reservation as the daughter, wife, and now widow of sheep farmers. She resided in a remote hogan in northern Arizona with her husband, Jimmy; 4 living children (3 others are deceased); 12 grandchildren, 15 great-grandchildren; 2 great-great-grand-babies; her mother; and several aunts (until their deaths). There she kept house, cared for children and elders, orchestrated religious ceremonies, practiced healing, wove rugs, and taught her offspring, in Dine language, the basics of being Navajo.

The family car was used on weekdays by her employed children. On Fridays, she was driven to the Flea Market in Tuba City, where she bought food supplies and remedies from other healers and socialized over mutton stew and fry bread with friends. Her father and husband were both singers and were often called to cure tribal members by touching or removing foreign objects from an afflicted body. Mrs. Mayflower herself was a specialist who prescribed herbs.

Margaret Mayflower's belief in Navajo spirituality and her self-esteem—which derived from being a productive, necessary person—were the major strengths that helped her cope with the deaths of her loved ones. Each time, she guided her family's grieving by observing traditional Navajo burial customs. For example, as a spiritual leader, she observed the taboo against talking about an approaching death, saw that the person died away from home, and had the hospital staff (never the family) "fix the body." Mourning, meditation, and positive thinking lasted 4 days; bathing, washing the hair, eating red meat, etc., were not allowed until the fifth day, when the spirit left. Only then could mourners shower, wash their hair, be holy again.

When her husband died, Mrs. Mayflower again followed the burial customs. But a combination of stress, obesity, and genetics brought on diabetes. Her love of fried foods kept her from maintaining a disciplined diabetic diet and added to her vascular problems. Finally her diabetes was so severe that she became insulin-dependent. Her noncompliance was ignored by her children, but she did receive regular monitoring by the IHS. Poor circulation to her legs resulted in nonhealing ulcers, and her right leg had to be amputated. She remained in a wheelchair in the hogan, isolated from her friends and unable to do many of her chores. In 1995, her left leg was amputated. Her usual good cheer disappeared.

Soon after that, her youngest son, Ashie, was killed in an automobile accident in Tempe. Rejecting Navajo ways, Ashie had left the reservation to attend Arizona State, married a white girl there, and seldom returned to the reservation. When Margaret learned that Ashie's new family did not observe Navajo burial customs, she became clinically depressed and did not eat well, sleep well, or feel well. She said her heart hurt. The family, in their words, consulted with "the holy people, to make her holy again, for Margaret, in her disharmony, had to find beauty in the springtime once more." A medicine man instructed her to sing chants as she was washed with herbs. She then meditated on positive thoughts for 7 days.

A month later, however, Mrs. Mayflower was still depressed and had lost 25 pounds. She cried most of the time. An IHS nurse asked Dawn A., a counselor, to see her. Mrs. Mayflower was resistant at first, but Mrs. A. established rapport by addressing her with a traditional Navajo phrase, "Hello my little grandmother." Soon Mrs. Mayflower responded, "Hello, my little granddaughter." They were off to a good start, but Dawn wasn't sure where to go next.

Lucy Longfeather, a Pueblo Indian From an Impoverished Environment, With Dementia But Good Family Support

Lucy Longfeather, age 79, lived her entire life on the Jemez Pueblo near Santa Fe, New Mexico. This small, compact village, a family-clan in itself, is chiefly agricultural. Mrs. Longfeather's life centered on child care, crafts, and housekeeping. Except for infrequent trips to the IHS in Santa Fe, she seldom left the pueblo, as she lacked transportation and had little facility in English. She spoke some Spanish, but she preferred her native Towa language, and that often created problems of communication with the outside world and even with her grandchildren.

Mrs. Longfeather married Jim Longfeather in 1936 and they later had four children. They lived in a terraced adobe with no modern conveniences; thus they had to carry water in, use an outhouse, and chop wood for heat.

Jim Longfeather died of cancer in 1987. Throughout his illness, the family had refused to talk about his condition or to touch him. He was buried in an unmarked grave without ado; but yearly, on November 1, All Souls' Day, the family members bring his favorite foods and celebrate with his spirit at the grave.

Mrs. Longfeather tried living alone in her home, relying on her granddaughter for transportation. She took meals at the tribal meal site, for sociability; or meals were delivered to her home when she took care of her great grandchildren, who were not eligible for the senior meal program. Most health care—monitoring her arthritis and cataracts—was provided on the pueblo and financed by Medicare, Medicaid, and the IHS. In 1990, her children noticed that she was confused at night and that her thinking was disorganized. She couldn't remember and was often lost.

The family moved Mrs. Longfeather into a daughter's new adobe ranch home, which had modern conveniences but was isolated and even further from the pueblo. Mrs. Longfeather was not comfortable there, even with a telephone and a television set. A large extended family resided there, and she tried hard to take care of the very young children while others were gone for many hours during the day. Her condition worsened. She was finally taken to the IHS hospital in Santa Fe with added presenting symptoms: impaired gait, incontinence, and confusion. A geriatric multidisciplinary team made a diagnosis of Alzheimer's-type dementia.

The patient's support system was also assessed. Dorothy G., the social worker, with the cooperation of Mrs. Longfeather's eldest son, invited the entire family for sessions. The tribal elder code was consulted, and although the sons were not expected to become caregivers, they were specified as spokespersons. Ms. G. told the family about a nursing home in the area staffed by a few American Indian nurses who spoke Towa. Native foods were offered, and Mrs. Longfeather could have day passes to celebrate powwows and feast days with the family. Ms. G. emphasized that Mrs. Longfeather would not have a male nurse, that no one at the nursing home would throw away any of her hair, etc.

Dorothy G. complimented the family members for their concern but pointed out that they could no longer help Mrs. Longfeather in the old way. She gave basic concrete information about the needs of Alzheimer's patients, levels of nursing care, and the dementia unit; and she stressed that Mrs. Longfeather was not crazy. She noted that there no caregivers' support groups were available.

The family resisted, saying that the pueblo would criticize them and talk about them. It was wrong to make such a decision. Dorothy G. reframed their concerns and said that it might look like they were neglecting their mother by *not* getting her the help she needed. She reminded them that they mustn't neglect their own children or their jobs but also that they could not leave their mother alone anymore. She suggested that they try a 30-day nursing home respite. She also offered to help them get permission for placement from their tribal council, and to get the medicine man's approval as well.

Joe Ramsey, an Urban AI From an Impoverished Environment with Alcoholism and No Family Support

Joe Ramsey, age 58, is the fourth son of a Chippewa father and an Oneida mother who left their reservations to find work in Milwaukee around 1920. Although very poor, the family survived the depression and other bad times—one son was killed in World War II and another in an automobile accident. The whereabouts of the third son are unknown. Both parents are now deceased. Mr. Ramsey was sickly as a child and had learning problems; he only finished ninth grade. His work history is one of many minimum-wage jobs and many layoffs. He now works as a janitor for a temporary agency and lives alone in a rented room. His income is at the poverty level, and he has no health coverage. He receives alcohol counseling and medical care from the Milwaukee Indian Community Health Center but gets no reservation benefits or governmental Indian-specific services. Twice weekly, he eats nutritious meals at St. John's.

Mr. Ramsey has been an alcoholic since age 14 and has burned out three families: his parents and brothers; his first wife, with three children; and his second wife, with four children. None of his living relatives keep in touch with him. He has been detoxified often and he has tried treatment and AA many times, but he could not relate to either. In 1993, he was diagnosed with heart disease and severe liver dysfunction and was told that his survival depended on immediate sobriety. He was referred to an Indian AODA program.

Frightened and worn out from binge drinking, Mr. Ramsey joined a support group and began counseling with Tom Evans, an Indian AODA specialist. After detox, they dealt with his lifelong feelings of helplessness and hopelessness, which had resulted in a pattern of apathy and projection. Mr. Ramsey blames his drinking and his irresponsibility on societal inequities. Tom Evans validates his feelings but points out that such projections only make recovery harder. Initial treatment goals focus on the "circle of recovery" in physical, emotional, mental, and spiritual areas. This includes finding and keeping a job, improved nutrition, and associating with nondrinkers. Now, counselor and client are working on returning to Native American spirituality practices, and to pride.

Chapter 4

The AI/AN Ethnic Lens

Looking through the ethnic lens of our first major ethnic category, we see the American Indian/Alaskan Native (AI/AN). Here, we will focus on identity, demographics, immigration and migration experiences, cultural values, and special issues, with an emphasis on the American Indian. It is hoped that the adding of the AI/AN Ethnic Lens onto the Gero Chi and the Gerocounseling Models will increase your understanding of these proud peoples. As you read, think of our fictional case examples and also of the AI/AN historical context.

Identity

The term American Indian/Alaska Native (AI/AN) designates aboriginal peoples of tribes and groups in the continental United States and Alaskan boundaries. Lately, Native American is used; but the term American Indian, which describes the indigenous peoples of North America, is still preferred by most AI/AN elders. Simply, the term that includes Indians, Eskimos, and Aleuts defines an ethnicity and a unique legal status in which AI/AN members maintain dual citizenship in the United States and in a specific tribal nation or subcategory. Special treaties therefore led to special rights, responsibilities, and relationships with the United States government. Such treaties also led to unfair treatment, broken promises, and minimal access to needed governmental services.

The peoples of this category are self-defined for census purposes; but to receive benefits and rights, an AI/AN must be officially enrolled on a tribal or reservation roster, reside on a reservation, prove one-fourth Indian blood (blood quantum), or show descent through genealogical documentation. Increasingly, over 50 percent of Indians marry non-Indians, causing later generations to lose benefits. A non-Indian wife or mother, or even children, may be denied eligibility for IHS benefits, for example.

There are approximately 333 Indian tribes, ranging in size from as few as four persons to over 150,000 (Navajos), speaking over 300 distinct languages plus English. Again, there are vast differences between and among each ethnic category and hence among tribes, as well as between individual elders. Let us look at some differences and commonalties.

Demographics

The 1990 Census reported 1.9 million AI/ANs, the smallest of all minorities in the United States, but many are uncounted. Some 114,453 (6 percent) are over 65 (compared with 27,851,973 whites over 65), of whom 9,205 are 85 or over (compared with 2,788,052 whites), with 73 men for every 100 women. The number of AI/AN elders grew 52 percent between 1980 and 1990, more than twice that of white or black older persons (AARP, 1990).

More than one-third of all Indians die before age 45, compared with 12 percent of the total population of the United States, and their life expectancy is eight years less than that of non-Indians. Indian old age is defined by social functioning (for example, grandparenting) or performance of ADLs, and this leads to inequities because most services for elders are based on chronology. Age requirements for services are lower only for tribal contractors on reservations.

The Choctaw Nation in Oklahoma has the highest percentage of persons over 65 (11.3 percent) followed by that state's Cherokees (10.4 percent). The largest nation, the Navajo, has only 4.8 percent (Stuart and Rathbone-McCuan, 1988). Overall, American Indians have the lowest median age of American minorities; because of this and their relative poverty, their multiple social and health problems, and their shorter life expectancy, the Administration on Aging (AoA) has designated them a priority group.

Less than 24 percent of AI/ANs live on the approximately 399 federally recognized reservations; 30 percent remain rural; and 46 percent live in urban areas. They live in every state, but most are in California, Oklahoma, Arizona, New Mexico, and Texas. Most live in California, where 90 percent are urban, 10,700 of whom are over 65 (McCabe and Cuellar, 1994). Elders usually live in three- or four-generational extended families.

Each tribe has its own language, culture, and history. The Navajo Tribe of Arizona and New Mexico is the largest—104,517 total, 5,000 over age 65, on 26,000 square miles—and has been the most researched. Following in population are the Cherokee, Dakota Sioux, Chippewa, Pueblo, Lumbee, Coctaw and Homa, Apache, Iroquois, and Alabama. Tribes in Alaska include the Eskimos, Aleuts, Athabascan, Tlingit, and Haida Indians.

Native Americans are the most impoverished of all ethnic groups. McCabe and Cuellar (1994) reported that many AI/AN elders on and off reservations are unemployed and estimated that only 23 percent to 50 percent of the employed are earning significantly less than the 66 percent of employed non-Indian elders in the general population. Less than one third reported having medical insurance, compared with three fourths in the total population. Eleven percent continue to work after age 65 compared with 12 percent of whites.

In 1990, the average income for an AI/AN male over 65 was $9,967, compared with $14,775 for comparable white males. The average income for AI/AN females over 65 was $6,004, compared with $8,297 for whites. Ten percent live below the official poverty level (AARP, 1990). Studies reveal low participation in Social Security programs, due to a dearth of knowledge about services, to problems of physical or linguistic access, and possibly to racism (McCabe and Cuellar, 1994).

Although there is much two-way traffic between reservations and urban areas, little is known about the urban Indians who constitute almost half of the AI/AN population. They are often called the invisible minority because they are underrepresented in the research on minority aging. Most, like Joe Ramsey's parents, left the reservation between 1920 and 1950 for economic betterment; but this has not occurred, and many are now at retirement age, with 81 percent reporting they do not plan to return to the reservation (Kramer, 1992). One third of urban Indians live in cities at poverty levels with other poverty-ridden relatives. Few have health insurance, and federally mandated health care provided by the Indian Health Service (IHS) expires after 180 days or residence off the reservation. Consequently, health clinics for urban Indians were created by the Indian Health Care Improvement Act in 1976.

The educational levels of AI/AN elders' are low; 12 percent had no formal education, compared with 2 percent of white elderly people. Seventy-eight percent of AI/AN elders on reservations did not complete high school. Many of them, discussed below, are called "boarding school elders."

Immigration and Migration Experiences

How and when AI/ANs immigrated to this continent is debated, though there is no disagreement that they were here first. Did they walk across the Bering Straits from Asia or was this once one total world mass that broke apart into continents? We know AI/ANs were nomadic peoples whose migrations enabled them to rotate crops and lands, find new food supplies, escape from enemies; and respond to the involuntary relocations imposed by European settlers. Since the 1920s, AI/ANs have migrated to urban areas for employment; recently, in what could be called a Pan-Indian renaissance, some are migrating back to reservation homelands. To the American Indian, the word *homeland* is sacred.

The story is that when European settlers arrived in the New World in the fifteenth century, Columbus, thinking he had found India, called the indigenous peoples Indians. They lived all over the continent, speaking many languages and pursuing different life styles. With a few exceptions, they were peaceful, resourceful peoples adapting successfully to their varied environments.

The American Indians traded commodities and shared knowledge about surviving in their vast wilderness with the European explorers and settlers who, despite such generosity, confiscated their homelands. The history of this relationship is a story of pillaging, warring, broken promises and treaties, unrealistic stereotyping, misunderstanding, manipulation, mocking, and mimicry. European Americans depicted AI/ANs as savages to be hunted, specimens to be scrutinized, infidels to be converted, barbarians to be civilized, hunters to be romanticized, spiritual sages to be imitated, and—in modern times—casino capitalists to be censured. Lately, many AI/ANs are indignant about "New Age" white people who imitate and exploit Indian ancestral spiritual traditions and icons.

It is no wonder that AI/ANs come to a negotiating table or to a health and social service agency with distrust. And it is no wonder that members of the dominant society approach AI/ANs with guilt. But, however understandable, both distrust and guilt are negative influences on any relationship and predictors of failure.

Despite the accounts in some American history texts, the early policy of the United States regarding AI/ANs was to eliminate them from areas where "civilized citizens" lived. AI/ANs were often violently removed from their own lands and forced into less desirable reservation areas. Many land-use treaties remain in the courts today, and it has been said that the mental health of AI/ANs is land-related.

The Indian schools, run by the Bureau of Indian Affairs (BIA) or private missionaries, aimed to Christianize and "civilize" Indians. Therefore, boundaries between teaching religion, morals, and school subjects were often blurred. The educational level was low, with only a few good teachers, who taught "at convenient and safe places among those tribes friendly to us" (Blanchard, 1983, p. 122). In 1969, the Kennedy American Indian Policy Review Commission reported that these conditions continued in some areas.

Most schools were boarding schools whose pupils had been almost forcibly enrolled at a very young age and made to discard their customary language, dress, and food for eight continuous years away from their tribal homes. Nonconsenting parents forfeited their food rations; and neither parents nor tribes had a voice in their children's educational programs. As a result, children were denied the specific education required to survive on the reservation.

Margaret Mayflower's children lived away, in Mormon homes in Utah; and Mary Banks attended a Catholic boarding school in South Dakota. For many, being exposed to new worldviews caused great identity problems that resulted in family disruptions, depression, and the use of intoxicants. Many lost personal self-esteem and Indian pride. Today AI/AN elders labeled "boarding school

Indians" still have conflicts with their own adult children who are trying to revive native pride. But despite the known traumatic effects of the boarding school movement, many grandchildren of today's elders continue to be sent away to foster homes, boarding schools, and other institutions to escape rural isolation and poverty.

Still, some communities are faring better with their children. In June 1995, a new million-dollar school, financed by Oneida casino revenues and architecturally designed to resemble a giant turtle— a tribal symbol—opened at the Oneida reservation in Northern Wisconsin. There, Indian children are taught by Indian teachers.

Attempts to assimilate AI/ANs into the dominant society were also part of the provision of health and social services. In the 1800s, the BIA provided staff physicians at most reservations and also provided food, shelter, and clothing. The Snyder Act (1921) and the Johnson O'Malley Act (1934) provided federal funds and supervision of social, educational, and health services to reservation Indians.

In 1924, all AI/ANs became United States citizens. This entitled them to all state and federal services and paved the way for their inclusion under the Social Security Act (1935), but few were eligible for Social Security because most worked in uncovered jobs.

The Older Americans Act of 1965, administered through the states, gave AI/ANs access to much needed health care, but not all states participated. Arizona, with a large Indian population, considered health care a "county responsibility," so the Indian Health Service (IHS) was the only resource Indians had. Arizona did not provide Medicaid until the mid-1980s.

The Indian Council on Aging was formed in 1981 to investigate Indian problems, but AoA-funded Title III programs continue to be underutilized by American Indian elders. Reasons cited by various authors are distrust, little outreach, cultural insensitivity, incompetent staffs, fiscal cuts, and the targeting of the neediest populations—which puts Indians into competition with other poor minorities. Also cited are the inefficiency and the politicization of BIA. Another problem is that the IHS Medicare-Medicaid geriatric contract care is available only to reservation Indians, but 50 percent of AI/AN elders live off reservations and thus are uncovered and vulnerable.

Long-term care is not considered a part of the IHS mandate unless skilled nursing care is needed, and even then, days are limited. There is also a dearth of AI/AN nursing homes. People requiring nursing home care, such as Margaret Mayflower, must travel far from family and tribe. Among the Navajos, an important cultural requirement is living within a region bounded by four sacred mountains; serious spiritual problems as well as isolation from family result when a placement is outside this holy area.

Limited resources put a strain on already overburdened families, creating a potential for elder abuse. Redhorse (1980) warned against stereotyping the AI/AN family in relation to long-term care: Filial piety exists, but many fragile families—struggling with poverty, with the needs of younger generations, and often with alcoholism—do not handle elder care adequately. There is elder abuse and neglect, and the oldest old are the most vulnerable.

Recommendations include continued promotion of self-determination, support of family participation in caregiving, local autonomy with financial aids, and training indigenous service providers. It has also been suggested that AoA Title VI programs be made available to off-reservation Indians, that Congress mandate the improvement of geriatric care under IHS, and that coordination and planning between BIA, HUD, and AoA be improved, giving AI/AN elderly people a priority (Stuart & Rathbone-McCuan, 1988).

Cultural Values

Most elders are proud of their cultural traditions. Their adult children, in a renaissance of Indian self-esteem, are also imparting this pride to their own children—the elders' grandchildren. This should help to unite generations. But as Curley wrote (1982), not all Indian elders fare this well. Many (like Mary Banks's parents) expected their children to return after their education, but the children were ashamed of their origins or were better off financially away from home. An Indian elder's special function is to pass on the cultural traditions, but when grandchildren live off the reservation or return for visits, this function is often thwarted by a language barrier which causes the elders to feel "isolation and a sense of failing to meet the criteria of a "successful" family.

To the AI/AN, traditions are not only reminders of the past but are axioms for life today. AI/ANs struggle to maintain a sense of wholeness while having to live in two conflicting cultures that expect opposite personal attributes. The dominant culture fosters competition, acquisitiveness, mercantilism, and individualism—traits that are antithetical to most AI/AN values. Indian children are given two paths of knowledge: One is tribal-specific and is internalized by emulating persons who exemplify certain values; the other that of the dominant society.

While AI/AN cultures are many and diverse, they share general themes. Many of their generic cultural values, such as those listed below, are misunderstood:

1 Sharing and generosity. Respect is shown for generosity and gift-giving. A prize won is a prize shared; it is called a "give away." This is a contrast with the majority culture, which respects individual acquisition and attainments. (As a result, AI/ANs are frequently depicted as poor and unmotivated to better themselves.)

2 Cooperation. Basic tenets are working together, getting along, and putting family and tribe over the individual. All life should be a harmonious whole rather than having an individual competitive focus. (Thus AI/ANs are sometimes seen as lacking goals.)

3 Noninterference. Observe; don't react; respect other's rights; don't meddle. Until recently, children were trained by the examples of multiple caretakers. (Thus AI/ANs have sometimes been seen as aloof, withdrawn, or overly permissive parents.)

4 Present. Often, the present reigns. Things get done in a natural order without deadlines or artificially imposed time frames. Life should be enjoyed first. (This relates to an old economy and to survival through rhythmic, circular patterns—in contrast to the clock-oriented, scheduled, punctual, long-term character of the dominant society. Thus the dominant culture may see AI/ANs as inefficient, laid back, and unmotivated.)

5 Orientation to the extended family. The strong extended family can total 200 or more blood relatives, clan members, etc., who have reciprocal interdependent relationships. (This is in contrast to the small nuclear family in the dominant society, which fosters independence.)

6 Respect for elders. Older persons are respected as teachers, historians, preservers of tribal culture, keepers of the lan-

guage, storehouses of knowledge of traditional cures, and critical members of society. Lessons in living have been passed on through elders' stories. (This too is in contrast to the dominant culture, where elders often receive little respect, childrearing is often done by nonrelatives, and knowledge and history are literate and linear.)

7 Harmony with nature. One is part of a greater whole, and balance and respect must exist between the living and non-living. (By contrast, the dominant society tends to separate self, society, and nature. The medicine person does not relieve symptoms as western medicine practioners do but restores harmony to the individual within a total universe. AI/ANs say that all living creatures have rights—an idea in contrast to the notion of controlling and dominating nature.)

8 Importance of tradition. Traditional ways that work are best; this contrasts with some other cultures' preference for new ways. But despite reliance on tradition, Indian societies have never been static; change and newness had a place if the old ways proved ineffective. Tribes share old and new skills, dress, music, and ceremonies. New songs are composed yearly.

Today there is a tendency to romanticize Indian culture. In the 1990s, people seeking a better life have discovered beauty and simplicity on the reservation, have found cures in Indian healing, have observed wisdom in Indian spirituality, and have developed formulas for saving the environment through Indian reverence of nature—while they collect and adorn themselves and their homes with Indian jewelry and art. Many do all this with respect and admiration, boosting Indian economies; others exploit "Indianness," profiting financially and callously as they market their versions of sweat lodges and dream catchers. Kramer (1990) pointed to blatant racist Indian stereotypes in certain American products: toys, costumes, greeting cards, and mascots of sporting teams that do not depict Indians as people. Some whites continue to make inaccurate assumptions and hold on to myths such as these:

1 *Myth:* Indians on reservations retain their culture; those off reservations deny it.
Fact: Urban Indian cultures vary considerably from main-

stream practices because AI/AN cultures are transmitted through family and other ethnic networks on or off the reservations.

2 *Myth:* When Indians get old, they retire to reservations.
Fact: Most urban elders "age in place" and do not return to reservations, so aging services are needed for them too.

3 *Myth:* American Indians, wards of the government, get "special services."
Fact: AI/ANS, are taxpayers, not governmental wards. But it is true that most health and social services are linked to reservations.

4 *Myth:* AI/ANs are a homogeneous culture, and all treat their elders the same.
Fact: AI/ANs vary in regard to appropriate behaviors such as treatment of elders. Nomadic Apaches and Athabascans, for instance, abandoned elders who were frail and no longer self-sufficient. In contrast, Pueblo farmers nurtured their elders.

We can learn much about a people by observing and partaking in their food customs, and food has always been an important part of AI/AN culture. For the holistic AI/AN, who often experienced shortages, food was valued as a sacred gift from nature and its uses followed specific spiritual, gender, and other cultural customs. Food was celebrated in ceremonies and was usually served according to a communal giveaway tradition—first to the most needy, elders, and children; then to men, the warriors; and finally to women. When I attended a lunch at an Oneida nursing conference, I was asked to begin the buffet procession as I, the elder and the guest, was to be honored by being "first served."

While Indian males gave firewood, clothing, and game, food was considered an important gift from women to men. Hopi women initiated marriage proposals by baking and placing a piki (a blue cornmeal cake) at a man's doorstep. Taking the cake inside signified acceptance.

Food was also used as medicine. Corn and cornmeal were said to prevent illness, to ease heart palpitations and rashes, to increase lactation, to relieve diarrhea and menstrual discomfort, and—among Zuni-women—to speed childbirth and prevent postpartum hemorrhaging. Indigenous plants such as agave, mint tea, and blood root were commonly used as healers. Also, certain foods, like cabbage, eggs, milk, and meat, were restricted during an illness. Some tribes forbade certain fish and huckleberries after childbirth.

Basic Indian staples were beans, corn, and squash, in addition to regional specialties. All, these crops, and the related methods of harvesting, preservation, and preparation, were shared with the settlers, who reciprocated with European products. Many "American" combinations followed, such as succotash, Boston baked beans, clam chowder, and Thanksgiving dinner.

Today, as poverty and fast foods have an impact on AI/ANs, their standard diet is high in carbohydrates, fat, and sodium and low in meat, eggs, and milk; as a result, many of their health problems are related to nutrition. Such new food habits, warned Kittler and Sucher (1989), indicate changes in ethnic identity. But while many AI/ANs have rejected traditional foods, others are reviving the foods of their ancestors in the new Indian movement.

EXERCISE

In your class or at home for yourself or family, plan and prepare an AI/AN meal. Bring in other cultural items, such as music, readings, etc. Or, if the timing is right, attend an Indian powwow and enjoy the ambience directly.

Issues: Sources of Pain and Pride

Issues stemming from racism and oppression of AI/ANs continue today. Most observers would agree that American public policies need revision and that Indian elders and their families require additional services. Understanding the history and cultural values of these peoples should pave the way for increased respect, empathy, and improved services.

Many people believe that the serious problems of AI/ANs—such as high levels of unemployment, substance abuse, poor health, poor nutrition, suicides, accidents, and domestic abuse—stem from a history of broken promises, pillaging, and poverty which have created a depressing picture of helplessness and hopelessness. All this affects AI/AN elders.

Alcohol abuse is probably the biggest problem for AI/ANs today.

Comparatively, their alcoholism rates are highest, and alcohol-related deaths at young ages are eight times higher among AI/ANs than any other category in the United States (Green, 1995, p. 222). Alcoholism is harder to treat among AI/ANs. Their drinking habits—often different from the general population—have been analyzed in various ways. Some see AI/AN alcoholism as a cultural construct, some as a reflection of continued poverty and lack of control, some as a genetic Indian disorder, some as a psychoactive substance necessary for religious rituals, some as a means of identifying with image of a hard western frontiersman, some as a saloon-oriented male bonding ritual, some as social interaction. As Morinis (1982) wrote, some also see drinking as "a symbol of exchange in an urban setting, one that deliberately inverts the standards of the larger society." To many AI/ANs, drinking is a treatment of choice.

But many people do not agree that alcoholism is an inevitable part of Indian life. A 10-year study of recovering Indians in a treatment program in Minnesota found that 7 out of 9 patients were sober for 2 years or longer; for these patients, abstinence was associated with stable employment, good economic and housing conditions, strong interpersonal relationships, and little depression (Westermeyer & Peake, 1983).

Elder abuse data are unavailable, but the fact that tribes target it for special services indicates that it is a problem. A study of a small Navajo community found that neglect was the most common form of abuse. Reasons cited were rapid onsets of dependency, mental health problems, and lack of income (McCabe & Cuellar, 1994).

Suicide rates of AI/ANs are the highest of all ethnic groups and are evidently linked to alcohol, poverty, and depression. Indian adolescents' rate of suicide is twice that of other ethnic adolescents. Among Indian young people at boarding schools, 23 percent report having attempted suicide. Suicides among AI/AN young people often occur in clusters of acquaintances who take hard liquor in lethal doses (Manson, Beals, Dick, & Duclos, 1989).

According to Green (1995), many people believe that this prevalence of suicide is a consequence of forced and incomplete acculturation. Others connect it to "deviant" marriage patterns in which lineages and clans are unequal and conflicting (Levy & Kunitz, 1987).

Indian gaming, officially recognized in 1994 when President

Clinton met with 542 tribal leaders to spell out the U.S. Supreme Court's 1987 ruling that liberated tribes, as sovereign nations, from most state gambling regulations. This has created a cultural and economic renewal. Called the "new buffalo economy," it is bringing Indians back to the reservations and is keeping others home by offering new employment opportunities. An article in the *New York Times* (Johnson, 1994) reported that in 1993 over 90 tribes had casinos, with total profits of more than $1 billion. In addition to jobs, casinos are financing new schools, housing, roads, and hospitals and are providing a startup for many new manufacturing and retailing businesses as well as educational and social services. The Indian Business Association, representing tourism and 5,000 Indian businesses, is booming; tribally run colleges grew from 1 in 1968 to 26 in 1994; and several tribal governments have established their own companies to drill for oil and gas or mine for coal on their own lands, netting billions of dollars of revenue.

Among the most lucrative gaming areas is the Mystic Lake casino in Minnesota, which paid 200 tribal members over $500,000 each in 1994. Running the largest casino—employing over 10,000 people—the 320-member Mashantucket Pequot tribe in Connecticut made even larger payouts to its members, as well as donating $10 million dollar to the Smithsonian Institution to help build the American Indian Museum.

Despite such windfalls, many critics deplore the casino craze, saying that it may lead to a cultural addiction among Indian gamblers. These critics also point out that not all of the profits go to Indians, that most of the casinos are managed by white-owned businesses, that some of the casinos have cheapened Indian dignity, and that the boom will not last—and then what?

Defenders of gaming hail it as the first thing that has worked in Federal Indian policy. They also stress that most profits are going into schools, social programs, and Indian infrastructure, and into new profit-making enterprises to take over if the interests in casinos end.

Such economic boosts are dramatic, considering that one third of the 2 million Indians in the United States still live in poverty—the proportion is even higher on reservations—and that Indians are the poorest American ethnic group. Not all of the tribes have gaming opportunities. These tribes continue to be in dire poverty, but the images of other prospering tribes can divert attention from their serious needs for services. Like the myth of the Asian American model minority, a number of success stories can work against less fortunate others in the same ethnic category. One third of the 2 million Indians in the United States still live in poverty and Indians are still the poorest American ethnic group. In South Dakota Indian country, unemployment exceeds 80 percent; on Navajo lands where shacks are common, it is between 30 and 40 percent (Johnson, 1994).

Strengths: Sources of Pride

But problematic issues tell only a part of the story; they are often highlighted to establish empathy and to get necessary policies and funding. In applying the Ethnic Lens to our understanding of AI/AN elders, we must not lose sight of the strengths springing from their cultures—that have enriched the dominant society. Nor should we forget the contributions of numerous AI/AN individuals, many of them now elderly.

To begin, though it seems almost trite to say this, AI/ANs shared their bountiful country with later settlers. They contributed to the general knowledge about health and survival skills through the introduction of nutrition, new foods, hygiene, and medicines too numerous to name.

The patterns, themes, colors, and artistry of Indian arts, crafts, and architecture influence how Americans live today, and Americans celebrate renowned Indian artists such as the painters Carl Gorman and Duke Sine; the dancer Maria Tallchief; the potters Maria Martinez, Teresita Naranjo, Helen Cordero, Mela Youngblood, and Alton Komatestewa; the silversmiths Atsidi Chon, Lanyade, and Lorenzo Hubbell; the jewelers Charles Loloma and Robert Sorrel; the carver Jose Astorga; the basketers Frances Manuel; and weavers such as Mae Jim—to name just a few!

AI/AN leaders such as Ada Deer and Wilma Mankiller have advanced the women's movement. AI/ANs such as Louis Bruce and John J. Matthews have succeeded in big business. Evelyn Yellow Robe and George Frazier have succeeded in their professions; Sequoya, Billy Mills, Russell "Big Chief" Moore, Edward "Wahoo" McDaniels, James Thorpe, and Charles Tinker have succeeded in sports. Famous contemporary entertainers include Buffy Sainte-Marie, Jay Silverheels, Ray Price, Keely Smith, Kay Starr, and of course Will Rogers. In government and the armed forces, there were Benjamin Reifel, Charles Curtis, Eli Samuel Parker, Peter McDonald, and Ira Hayes—all of whom rose to the top. Rosa Minoka Hill was the second female physician in the United States. AI/AN history buffs revere heroes such as Geronimo, Tecumseh, Crazy Horse, Sitting Bull, and countless others.

The Ethnic Lens should include these magnificent contributions—not necessarily to make the dominant culture feel guilty, but to increase respect and admiration for these outstanding American citizens. They are either today's American Indian and Alaska Native elders or today's heritage of the elders.

EXERCISE

Think about Mary Banks, Margaret Mayflower, Lucy Long-feather, and Joe Ramsey, and any AI/AN elders you may know. Could any of the historical events listed at the beginning of this chapter have affected their lives? How? Consider the dimensions of the Ethnic Lens. What part might any of these dimensions play in their present problems?

Chapter 5

The AI/AN Gero Chi Lens

For most AI/ANs, "gero" begins before age 45. During middle age, they experience the physical, emotional, and social declines characteristic of the general American population at age 65 and over. Typically, age 45 is "old" on reservations; in cities, "old" is age 55. Among AI/ANs, aging is defined by social and physical functioning, not chronology (National Indian Council on Aging, 1981). We must make these and other important corrections when we overlay the AI/AN Ethnic Lens on the Gero Chi Lens.

The Self-System

Our next adjustment is in the self-system. The independent individual at the core of the dominant culture's model must be altered to become the unique but interdependent person in a family, clan, and tribe. Here, family or clan is the basic unit.

Self-Concept

It is said that in many AI/AN cultures, there is no hierarchical order of life; insects share existence on a par with humans. All living things have a place in the natural order.

With an emphasis on interdependence, AI/ANs usually divided labor and social responsibility along generational and gender lines. Each clearly defined secular or religious task gave a sense of one's unique part in the world order and of one's own unique worth. This is unlike the individualism of the dominant culture, which one may depart from a norm. Here, as Blanchard wrote, "uniqueness becomes the refinement of life" (1983, p. 117).

Self-Esteem

A recent resurgence of tribalism is providing more group esteem and self-esteem. Well-being is tied to a sense of selfhood accomplished through adherence to a historic culture and transmitted through family interaction. A relationship between land and emotional well-being (self-esteem) is noted.

Gender is important in AI/AN societies. Tribes can be patriarchal, matriarchal, or egalitarian. Many still have practices, dictated by tribal economic and social needs or preferences, believed to influence the sex of an unborn child. For example, the Pueblos preferred females; Apaches, males. The marital picture of AI/ANs is similar to that of whites; most men over 65 are married, and a larger number of older women are widowed. Consequently, older single women are more at risk of poverty.

Females

Many clans trace their ancestry through matrilineal descent, and the female traditionally performs the necessary duties of preserving social organization and regulating matters of marriage, adoption, and discipline. Today over one third of AI/AN families are female-headed and "American Indians are characterized by a high fertility rate, a large percentage of out-of-wedlock births, and a strong role for women" (U.S. Bureau of the Census, 1990).

Males

Matrilineal descent sometimes presents problems for AI/AN males if a bridegroom is unfavorably regarded by members of the wife's lineage or clan. Marrying into a wife's lineage means that her brothers have more power over the household, religious ceremonies, songs, and sometimes land use. Green wrote that such stress has been great in "small, face-to-face communities," especially for members of more egalitarian tribes like the Hopis (1995, p. 227).

Romanticized history portrays AI/AN males as brave, proud hunters, but today's data on poverty, high unemployment, alcoholism, and high suicide rates indicate that their pride has been injured. Joe Ramsey is an example.

Spirituality

Most AI/ANs worship as the dominant society does, but their religious practices may be influenced by earlier cultural roots. AI/AN spirituality is also tied to beliefs about health, disease, and healing. With Navajos, for example, the sacred core of religion is a healing system that stresses causes and prevention rather than symptoms. It is believed that contact with spirits of the dead is dangerous and can cause illness. Patients prefer to die in hospitals so that medical personnel can handle the corpse and arrangements and burials are done quickly and not close to home.

Navajos use six healers: (1) a positive medicine person who can only heal, (2) a positive-negative medicine person who heals but can also cause illness through evil spells and witchcraft, (3) a "divine diagnostician" who discovers causes and cures but cannot heal, (4) a specialist, like Margaret Mayflower, who prescribes herbs and sets bones, (5) a sacred medicine person who heals the soul, and (6) a singer who cures by touching and removing foreign objects from the body (Bean, 1976).

Are medicine men and women common today? At the Oneida reservation, I was told about a medicine person who administers to north-central tribes, although his whereabouts are guarded so that he is not abused through overuse. On the Navajo reservation, the medicine person is more commonplace, is consulted regularly, and often works side by side with mainstream physicians. Remedies for various medical problems are sold at the Friday Tuba City flea market.

Psychosocial Tasks

One way to learn about your AI/AN elder client is by considering traditional child-rearing methods. Such methods were used in the early socialization of your client and help to explain who he or she is now. Many remain today, but others were modified with acculturation, perhaps even creating intergenerational differences. They are also important to know about because help with child rearing has usually been assigned to elders. The Gero Chi Lens uses Erikson's psychosocial model (1950).

Hope (Trust versus Distrust)

In AI/AN societies, as in other interdependent societies, the education and training of the young was a shared community responsibility and relationships extended beyond bloodlines. Multiple caretakers, including many elders, maintained a child-centered system. The AI/AN child communicated with and received stimulation from many people. Mature language was fostered from the start.

Each child was important and central to tribal life. Since infant mortality was high, a healthy child was cherished and children symbolized renewal and immortality—also, children held the promise of becoming future providers and caretakers of the old.

Will (Autonomy versus Shame)

AI/AN children were socialized nonverbally through observing others' expectations and through imitating older children. They developed freely, with no emphasis on the timing of tasks, and were given freedom to act out feelings among themselves. To an outsider, their behavior appeared chaotic, but it did not reflect a lack of parental authority. Using an interpersonal process instead of punishment, elders could be stern, demanding, and rigorous.

Because AI/AN children were encouraged to be sensitive to the opinions of others, they did not always develop the defense mechanisms and habits necessary for adaptation to the dominant culture, and they were more vulnerable to criticism.

Purpose (Initiative versus Guilt)

Much attention was given to the sexual identification of AI/AN children through instruction and gender-related activities. Early on, communication patterns made gender distinctions; boys were instructed by males, girls by females.

Competence (Industry versus Inferiority)

Little is known about the distinct learning patterns of AI/ANs. Early learning was filled with shapes, colors, and ceremonies.

AI/AN children were encouraged to relate to their world and to have community learning experiences in close contact with others who praised, guided, urged, warned, and scolded but—most importantly—respected (Blanchard, 1983). But the learning experiences of boarding-school children, forced into alien environments, denied them their own and their community's integrity. Today, AI/ANs continue to be more successful in learning in early childhood when teaching is based on tribal language.

AI/AN children were taught to be cooperative, not competitive; this made it difficult for them to succeed in the competitive world of the dominant culture. Close living arrangements, as in modern-day pueblos (which caused problems for Lucy Longfeather when dementia set in), require the learning of tension-reducing behaviors.

Fidelity (Identity versus Diffusion)

AI/AN cultures place great reliance on ancient family and tribal histories; but when adolescents were forced into foreign environments, their sense of community was compartmentalized. Self-redefinition was necessary creating self-diffusion at a critical time when the opposite—self-integration—was needed. Some, who had well-established tribal and family support systems, were able to integrate Indian skills with those of the dominant society. Others, like Mary Banks, denied their identity and needed a rebirth later.

In 1983, more than 30,000 Indian children were still enrolled in schools hundreds of miles away from home, separated from strong, sensitive AI/AN role models. Older children with similar discontinuity patterns were their support systems and were often unfit, unqualified teachers. T. Wilson (personal communication, 1997) pointed out that while rural isolation is a major factor in the continuing use of boarding schools, another incentive for parents is that they cannot afford to feed and clothe children at home.

Other Indian children learn in economically depressed communities where abuse of intoxicants is prevalent. Unprepared to survive, many are forced to work outside the reservation, where they often become part of another culture of poverty, unemployment, and drugs.

Brother-sister and cousin relationships are close among teenagers when both material and spiritual exchanges of assistance are needed.

Love (Intimacy versus Isolation)

This is the young person's period of embarking on work and love relationships. But many youthful AI/ANs are not prepared to hold jobs that offer a living wage, and unemployment rates are high. For a lucky few, reservations generating wealth through casinos offer jobs.

Although young girls are taught to be modest, sexual relations are common at an early age, resulting in many teenage pregnancies. Alcohol, a substance condoned by many societies, helps to blur the sense of emptiness. Drugs too become habitual.

Marriages that are within a tribe's accepted boundaries do better than those that link socially unequal clans or communities. Deviant marriages expose families to community stigmatization, putting them at the highest risk of alcoholism & suicide (Levy and Kunitz, 1987).

Care (Generativity versus Stagnation)

AI/ANs are raised with a custom of giveaways, so generosity is a common value. Therefore, this period is not difficult for most. I was repeatedly impressed with the generosity and hospitality afforded me as I did research for this chapter. The downside is that when too much is expected of financially poor families, or when these families are overburdened, they have problems of child abuse and elder abuse.

Wisdom (Integrity versus Despair)

Traditionally, the AI/AN elder was regarded as the tribe's bastion of wisdom—commanding respect and obedience in the family, clan, or tribe. For AI/ANs, aging has been a proud station in life, offering special rights and also particular responsibilities that kept elders active and engaged in meaningful activities. Some of these values have become watered down with increased assimilation. How such values will evolve in the future remains to be seen.

The Subset Systems

The Ethnic Lens, layered onto the Gero Chi Lens, also implies changes in the biopsychosocial systems of our AI/AN geroclients and their families.

The Biological System

While tribes vary in health practices, traditional beliefs about health prevail among many AI/AN elders, despite efforts to modify them. Today, many combine medical treatments of their traditional culture with those of the dominant culture, often going to an "Amerindian healer" before or while they see a western physician.

Healing is more than biological; it is also sacred. Many AI/ANs believe that health results from harmony between person, nature, and universe. Healing involves restoration of that harmony with supernatural or other forces whether the problem is internal (e.g., a violation of a taboo) or external (e.g., a broken bone). As a holistic approach to the physical, psychological, social, and spiritual worlds, healing involves mind, body, and soul.

If religious ceremonies prove ineffective in healing—as with blindness, deafness, and crippling diseases—the case is considered hopeless and ignored. This attitude, plus the high cost of western medicine, often leads to medical noncompliance, which is especially dangerous to diabetics and to patients requiring specific regimes (Yee, 1991).

Health Status

The IHS reported a rise in life expectancy from 67 in 1980 to 71.1 in 1990. Since 1940, when the life expectancy was 51, the leading cause of death changed from infectious diseases to chronic and alcohol-related diseases and injuries.

IHS data, based on 60 percent of the total population, also revealed excessive death rates among AI/ANs: 87 percent excess deaths before age 45, compared with 39 percent for blacks. These were attributed (in order) to unintentional injuries, cirrhosis, homicide, suicide, pneumonia, and diabetes—all possible consequences of risky lifestyles. Alcohol abuse is a prime cause of premature deaths for both sexes, and along with poor eating habits, it creates nutritional deficits. Deaths from diabetes are especially high among AI/ANs, who are 10 times more likely than whites to develop diabetes. Obesity is another major health risk.

The 10 leading causes of death among AI/ANs over 65 are in order (1) heart disease, (2) malignant neoplasms, (3) cerebrovascular disease, (4) pneumonia and influenza, (5) diabetes mellitus, (6) accidents, (7) chronic obstructive pulmonary disorder (COPD), (8) nephrotic diseases, (9) chronic liver disease–cirrhosis, and (10) septicemia (Indian Health Service, 1991).

As noted, poor nutrition is a serious problem. Federal nutrition programs were established under Title III-C and Title VI of the Older Americans Act of 1965, but follow-up studies are not readily available. Kramer (1990) reported a lack of access to both programs for many persons.

Vehicle accidents and falls are the major causes of hospitalizations among older AI/ANs. Fifty-nine percent of older AI/ANs have reported limited functioning—a number higher than that for any other ethnic group. While urban Indians are a population at risk, particularly for cardiovascular disease and diabetes, they responded with generally positive self-assessments of health in a multisite survey. Few except those with multiple disabilities reported functional problems (Kramer, 1990).

Service Barriers

Public policy has created some barriers to health services, discussed in the previous section. Other barriers include mutual misunderstanding, distrust of cultural norms and etiquette, lack of access, and shortages of trained AI/AN service providers.

The Psychological System

In a study of some 58 elderly American Indians in the Midwest, 64 percent reported life satisfaction and mental health above a midpoint score for congruence, mood, zest, and fortitude. They did not equate life satisfaction with material things but rather associated it with good hearing and vision, access to other people, and not being lonely (Johnson, Cook, Kelleher, Kentopp, & Manniein, 1986).

Most traditional AI/ANs believe that mental illness is caused by an imbalance in the natural order created by disruptions in human relationships, by natural disasters, or by undesirable influences from within or outside the tribe. Sometimes such events are viewed positively, if they lead to an improved understanding of the balance of life or the nature of the world and one's relationship to it.

Some indicators point to serious mental health problems in the AI/AN population. Unlike black elders, older AI/ANs report considerable worry and a feeling of being worse off financially. Depression is the mental problem most frequently diagnosed among AI/AN elders (Manson, Shore, & Bloom, 1985). For elders, other illnesses frequently diagnosed are schizophrenia, neurosis, personality disorders, and organic brain syndrome. "Evidence indicates that those who are least acculturated and maintain a tribal identity tend to have fewer problems" (Markides & Mindel, 1987).

Accurate data on dementia are unavailable, probably because there is no reporting system and also because AI/ANs have a greater tolerance for deviant behavior and are thus more accepting of early forms of dementia.

It is said that to compete in the dominant culture AI/ANs must be "white outside and Indian inside." This requires inclusion and reconciliation of different values, such as "Anglo" competitiveness and assertiveness, with a strong Indian value system. It also requires sufficient ego strength, good role models, and reinforcement from family and peers.

Today's AI/AN elders often cannot live up to previous role models because the status and tasks of elders have changed and lessened. The current educational system of their grandchildren, for example, can often be a source of conflicting values and expectations. Also, elders cannot pass down their culture when language differences exist in the family. Different urban norms are confusing to reservation elders who move out to find a "better life." Families are often overburdened with fiscal and psychological demands, and elder abuse (either direct abuse or neglect) occurs. Policies and programs for long-term care in and outside of institutions and on or off the reservation are lacking, and culturally specific nursing homes are often far from the patient's community. All of these factors, and more, create barriers to maintaining mental health.

The Sociological System

Because the AI/AN social order was not hierarchical, no aberrations existed. For example, gays lived unquestioned in Indian societies simply because "they existed;" in fact, homosexuality was often institutionalized. Pressure for conformity, when it was exerted at all, was based on reciprocal expectations of both individuals and the group, providing security for everyone.

Family Systems

Vertical and horizontal families (often clans consisting of many households) prevail in most AI/AN cultures. Clans are groups of families or households that trace descent through the head of the house from a common matrilineal or patrilineal ancestor.

Grandparents and older namesakes, preservers and teachers of tribal history and custom, become the active superegos of the clan. They can set standards of discipline and have the right to express approval or disapproval of parental behavior. "For most white Americans, the dream of retirement and the so-called golden years is independent living and self-sufficiency. The essence of Indian elderhood is grandparenting" (Green, 1995, p. 234). Grandparents are still considered the most knowledgeable members of the tribe, and they transmit tradition and sensibility to the next generation.

Five distinctive American Indian grandparenting styles were identified by Weibel-Orlando (1990). The most common was that of the cultural conservators, who take in their grandchildren for lengthy periods of time to instruct them in Indian ways—as Mary Banks's mother did. The style next most frequently cited was that of fictive unrelated grandparents with good reputations for grandparenting, who free employed young mothers.

As mentioned, brothers and sisters are usually very close. Uncles are important; and cousins, even second cousins, are often as close as siblings in white nuclear families.

Caregiving for Elders

A study of white and AI/AN caregivers found more expressions of control, anger, and guilt among whites and greater loss and passive forbearance among AI/ANs. Both groups saw preventive health measures as a responsibility of outside providers (Strong, 1984). On a Hopi reservation, I· learned that Indian caregiving was facing many of the same issues as the dominant culture. Usually, only one daughter is chosen for this role, even if siblings are available. If this daughter works outside the home—as is often the case—she may experience "caregiver burnout."

Tasks of Aging

Do AI/AN elders and their families face the same tasks as people in the dominant and other cultures? Yes, for the most part. The efficient use of medical, social, and emotional supports, adjustment to declining physical strength and health, maintenance of satisfactory living arrangements, coping with retirement and financial changes, assumption of new community responsibilities, revision of relationships, and adjustment to loss of significant others—these are not only tasks but should also be rights.

In some cases, however, the Ethnic Lens will modify the task of achieving or maintaining independence and asserting control over one's life. Many AI/ANs value interdependence over independence, and so they may leave important life decisions to the family-clan-tribe as well as or even instead of the individual.

Added to these tasks of aging should be the harmonious reconciliation of the ethnic and dominant cultures so that AI/AN elders can spend their final days feeling comfortable in their own culture and can achieve integrity instead of succumbing to despair. But deciding whether and how much to acculturate, assimilate, or neither is, of course, up to the individual.

EXERCISE

Think again about the case examples at the beginning of this section. After layering the Ethnic Lens onto the Gero Chi Model, what knowledge about AI/ANs do you now have that deepens your understanding of these four AI/AN elders and their families? What additional information do you need?

Chapter 6

AI/ANs and Gerocounseling

Now we will layer the Ethnic Lens onto the Gerocounseling Model to determine what counseling theories and methods, if any, need to be altered to accommodate AI/AN elders and their families. As you recall, gerocounseling includes some generic counseling principles and techniques and also the special handling of assessment, goal-setting, modalities and interventions, and terminations that are most appropriate for elders' issues.

Ethno-Generic Gerocounseling

Ethics Skills

Three ethical principles guide all good counseling: autonomy, beneficence, and fidelity. Each should be maintained at all times unless there are overriding factors, such as a risk of suicide. At times, however, the needs and values of the dominant society's biomedical or social ethics are in conflict with an ethnic elder's value system.

It is therefore critical to learn immediately about the ethics and meaning systems of the elders and families with whom you work. This task is easier if you are of the same ethnic background, but even then you will find variances. McCabe and Cuellar (1994) cited an example.

> Tribes and villages/groups may have varying beliefs concerning death, dying, social justice, autonomy, beneficence, and confidentiality. From one perspective, the traditional Navajo point of view concerning death and dying is seen as a part of the circle of life. Although death is a natural occurrence not to be interfered with, hope of continued life must never be omitted. The Navajo have defined principles of autonomy, beneficence, confidentiality, and social justice according to their culture. These principles have not been used to justify the activities associated with biomedical ethics as the Western culture has seen fit to do. (p. 33)

If you are Anglo, you may have to adjust some of your own ideas as you interact with interdependent extended AI/AN families. For example, elder clients may expect that any health issue will be discussed with family members and will not be the sole decision of the patient. You must avoid imposing your own values regarding advance directives, self-determination, independence, time orientation, etc.

Such accommodations can sometimes be frustrating. I have attended several American Indian conferences, and at one an elder presenter spoke way beyond the program's specified time limit. It was explained later that, "In our culture, an elder is not to be interrupted; the program will take care of itself." While this was an honorable idea (and the program did take care of itself), there were hungry participants in the audience, there was an angry food service staff, and the program coordinators were tearing out their hair.

If you have an appointment with an AI/AN and a member of that client's extended family or clan stops by requesting help, your client will probably give priority to the family member's need and miss your appointment (Wilson, 1983). So you must be prepared for different experiences and adjust your expectations accordingly.

It is also important to avoid stereotypes of what an AI/AN is like. All elders are different, and all AI/ANs are different too—especially in degree and form of assimilation or acculturation.

For example, in January 1996, I drove far into the Hopi Reservation at Second Mesa, Arizona, to interview a Hopi ombudsperson. I was a stranger in the area, and I miscalculated my driving time, so I was an hour late. My anxiety was allayed when I remembered "Indian time," telling myself, "She won't mind." But while she was tactful about my tardiness, I learned that this Hopi reservation woman, who lived on top of the mesa, was also a sophisticated alumna of Arizona State—an MSW—who had lived and worked all over the world and observed "regular time," thank you. It was evident that my lateness had messed up her day's schedule.

Relationship Skills

Owing to their long history of ill-treatment, AI/AN elders are often fearful and suspicious of health and social service bureaucracies. Thus ethnogerocounseling may have to begin with a gentle, nonconfrontational exploration of the client's feelings of distrust toward both native and nonnative professionals. Many AI/ANs have learned to just stay away or make a nonresponse as a means of coping with distrust. On the other hand, your AI/AN client or family may be very appreciative of your help and may want you to share in a giveaway, or even share a giveaway with you because you are now part of their lives. Refusing would be rude.

Unsuccessful non-Indian providers sometimes defend themselves by saying, "Indians do not care about prevention or services," but this has not been true historically. Often, AI/ANs have stayed away from services simply because agencies were of poor quality—understaffed, underfinanced, or overutilized.

Communication Skills

A rule of thumb is to follow the client's lead in nonverbal communication. Ask about behavior you don't understand. For example, eye contact between a young person and an elder may be considered disrespectful or even insulting. People in some tribes use rapid eye blinking to signal one another. Shyness and silence may be meant to convey respect. American Indians talk less, observe more, and listen attentively.

With many AI/AN people, I was told, it is good to talk in "the beauty way"—that is, positively. This is especially important in explaining advance directives such as living wills or durable power of attorney or requirements of the Patient Self-Determination Act (passed by the IHS in 1992). A highly regarded Navajo medicine man commented,

> In my practice, when I'm working with the patient, I am very careful of what I say, because any negative words could hurt the patient. So, with Western medicine, a doctor could be treating a patient, and he can mention death, and that is sharper than any needle. Therefore, with the tongue that we have, we have to be very careful of what we say at the time and point we're treating the patient. (Carrese and Rhodes, 1995, p. 828)

Use of interpreters is important but problematic. Sometimes AI/AN interpreters do not understand your issues and therefore find it hard to convey information about medical matters or social services, or they themselves may not be fluent. Conflicts can arise if an interpreter is a family member and is forbidden by the culture to discuss certain subjects.

On the Hopi reservation (in 1996), Aurelia Nehoitewa told me that her knowledge of the language was indispensable to her work with Hopi elders, and that her return to the reservation had helped her to relearn her culture. After living around the world with the United States military, she and her family had some important adjustments to make at first, but they now enjoy living on the mesa.

If Nehoitewa had cultural mores to relearn, what do you need for more cultural competence? For example, do you expect an easy verbalization of feelings with people (such as AI/ANs) who may find this behavior alien or even rude? What other forms of communication must you learn about? Sometimes it is a matter of trial and error, as in the following account of a physical fitness study involving prescribed weight loss for Native Americans in Nevada:

> Some of the tribal members who participated in formulating the program were shy and quiet, thus slowing planning efforts. . . . We were advised that elderly Indians did not like being touched, thereby obviating some of the measurement techniques. They also indicated that language barriers, between younger tribal members who were no longer proficient in their native tongue, might impact on interviews with Indian elders. This group also advised us that Indian elders may be suspicious of our intentions and the indigenous inter-

views. During the educational phase, we soon learned that lectures and discussions are best delivered, and received through visual teaching techniques which incorporate demonstration and animation (Greenhouse & Dodson, n.d., p. 1)

Learning and communicating about culturally different relationship skills should be reciprocal. Non-AI/AN professionals can appreciate the work patterns of indigenous providers: Although these providers sometimes do not have professional degrees, most are finely tuned to the needs and expectations of their clients. Non-AI/ANs must not impose their own work habits or challenge local procedures that they don't understand.

On the other hand, new AI/AN ethnic professionals can also learn some tried-and-true practices from the dominant culture. For example, in 1994 and 1995 I heard two different AI elder abuse counselors say that they had increased their effectiveness with "their people" because they offered very long weekend and evening sessions and did not stick to modern-day professionally prescribed time limits as members of the dominant culture did. Both, however, admitted that they were resigning after a year, owing to "burnout."

Ethnogerocounseling Assessment

Your first assessment goal should be to learn about the geroclient's values, meaning system, and issues of cultural identity or conflict. It is also important to understand your clients' health belief model. According to Manson (1994), when a person with one worldview comes into contact with another worldview, misunderstanding usually results. Experiences of health, illness, and suffering are not only perceived differently but verbalized differently through idioms and metaphors.

To many, for example, the heart, not the mind, is the center where the essence of self resides. In discussing depression, an AI/AN may describe a "heavy heart" instead of the usual endogenous symptoms. Perceived underlying causation and timing may also differ; AI/ANs may think of the problem in terms of "spiritual pollutants" or may think the symptoms are not abnormal at all but merely a part of "life's problems."

But another word of caution! An American Indian provider told me that while you will want to know what traditional medicine is being practiced, the direct question "Do you go to a medicine man?" would be considered improper. In an audiotape made by Manson and paraphrased below, a clinician interviewed a Musko-gee grandmother to learn more about her medical problem.

> I am full of sugar, Gramma told me. . . . The dr. told me what happened in my body. A bad spirit came and I was told ways to take care of it. But I have always been afraid of white folks and things they have around their necks. I felt I had to be another person with the doctor and was taught to just respectfully listen and not ask questions. I believed I was full of sugar and periodically I go to the Medicine Man but now he is scarce. He recommended teas, prayers, roots to chew. He said it would not go away but get better. He was willing to be one of the family, respect and caring, and I let him into my family. (Manson, 1994).

What is the family system like for this woman and other AI/AN clients? In your assessment, do not expect it to resemble the nuclear family of the dominant society or other contexts. Metz (1991) wrote that an Indian family is almost indefinable in the English language because the family is not a part but the whole of Indian life; it cannot be separated from spirituality, art, music, respect for the earth, the decision-making process, medicine, and animals.

Ho (1987) and Burlingame (1995) have recommended a geno-gram to facilitate family assessments. Genograms can serve many purposes. As graphic devices for mapping family history and rela-tionships, they also help to evaluate intangibles such as affect, memory, and orientation. They can help you establish initial rap-port in both individual and family sessions and help you introduce the "life review."

You will also want to assess the degree of assimilation or accul-turation of your AI/AN clients. Some, like Lucy Longfeather and Margaret Mayflower, have minimal contact with the dominant cul-ture; others, like Joe Ramsey, do not identify with tribal values at all. Mary Banks and others move between two worlds; they want the right to chose but may still work to advance their tribes.

Such assessments lead to understanding of geroclients' and fam-ilies' identity, their fear of failure and ridicule, and their exposure to successful AI/AN role models. Does a client feel alienated from tribal and extended-family values? What are the differences within a group?

To help with this assessment, Zitzow and Estes (1981) developed a typology for conceptualizing this varied AI/AN category. A two-point continuum was proposed with "heritage-consistent Native American" (HCNA) at one pole and the "heritage-inconsistent Native American" (HINA) at the other.

The HCNA has a basic AI/AN culture characterized by an extended-family orientation, involvement in tribal religion and culture, a reservation education, American Indian social interactions, knowledge about the AI/AN culture, a low priority for materialistic goals, and the use of shyness or silence to indicate respect. In counseling HCNAs, the goal may be to help individuals develop skills for coping with the dominant society. Issues may include:

1. Security is limited to reservation, tribe, family.
2. Indian and nonverbal language precedes English.
3. Socialization is comfortable only with other Indians.
4. Academic learning skills are underdeveloped.
5. Conflict occurs between learning and reservation values.
6. Failure and its impact on family-tribe are a big concern.
7. Long-term goals are of lesser importance.
8. Suppression of emotions is regarded positively.
9. Indecisiveness may result from governmental paternalism.
10. The dominant culture's expectations may be foreign.

The HINA's lifestyle is similar to the dominant American culture, but there also are many overlaps with native culture. In counseling HINAs, the goal may be to examine and solve conflicts of values and self-identity. Issues may include:

1. There is denial and a lack of ethnic pride.
2. Pressure to adopt the majority's values is seen.
3. Guilt over being removed from the culture is present.
4. Negative views about Native Americans exist.
5. A lack of support and belief system is evident.

You will also assess the client's support system. After having already looked at that in terms of tribal and family supports, you should also know about the relationship between the local, state, and federal social service and health institutions of the dominant community and the indigenous people you are serving. What interpersonal behaviors are necessary and seen in these cross-cultural settings?

Goals of Ethnogerocounseling

Counseling goals for HCNAs and HINAs are described above. Good goals depend on good assessments. By now you must have a clear picture not only of your unique client, family, clan, and tribe and their culture but also any intragroup differences. As noted, many intermarriages exist today, and levels of acculturation differ widely. Appropriate goals will also be different for an AI/AN living on a reservation compared with one living in an urban setting who has few traditional beliefs.

Goals dictate your counseling style. Because AI/ANs are not socialized to express feelings easily, they can't be expected to talk about sensitive subjects until trust is established. According to Trimble and LaFramboise (1985), most counselors concur that their goals and processes should involve the family, but this can create problems:

> As can be expected, group consensus in goal-setting is time-consuming, but an American Indian family has a flexible time orientation. The family can wait patiently for a group decision and will experience no urgency in completing certain tasks required of each family member for change. Hence, the time-limited and goal-directed mentality of the therapist may need modification when working with an American Indian family. (p. 130)

Modalities of Ethnogerocounseling

Various counseling modalities are used with AI/ANs, but in all modalities special outreach efforts should be made in the daily environment of the family or clan.

In family sessions, the culturally sensitive ethnogercounselor is encouraged to involve everyone important—the client's family, clan chief, traditional healer, etc. Home visits are imperative. In planning, remember that the structure of an AI/AN extended family differs from that of a nuclear family in the dominant culture. AI/ANs have a strong sense of family both vertically (grandparents, parents, children) and horizontally (siblings, cousins); and grandparents and older namesakes operate as active superegos who intervene if they disapprove of parental behaviors. Family counselors are advised to include grandparents in sessions about younger family members and to offer some separate sessions to children or adult children, because they must not speak negatively in front of their mothers. "Whenever possible, use a family treatment or group treatment modality" (Zitzow and Estes, 1981, p. 138).

In recommending family therapy as the treatment of choice for AI/ANs, Ho (1987) advised that while therapy with American Indians is based on a list of presumed Indian values such as harmony with nature, cooperation, and a present time orientation, don't limit it to that. The counselor should move on to the cultural relevance of interventions and should be alert to cultural values underlying choices and actions. Since group interdependence usually takes precedence over personal needs, the main goal should usually be to reestablish harmony within the family. This requires less psychodynamics and more group consensus about what needs to be done.

Ethnogerocounseling Interventions

How can we modify our interventions to fit AI/ANs? On this point, writers vary. Trimble and LaFramboise (1985) wrote that client-centered approaches are wrong because Indians prefer a more active, directive, problem-solving approach. But Wise and Miller (1983) saw a direct approach as confrontational, and stressed that it is important not to force a client to reveal sensitive subjects until trust is established. Sue and Sue's (1990) approach stresses timing: An appropriate combination of client-centered counseling with behavioral strategies may be very effective for traditional Indians, but bicultural families may do better with customary counseling methods. So, as with all geroclients and their families, the best interventions may be based on an eclectic one—"different strokes for different folks."

What are some of the "different strokes"—alternative counseling approaches and interventions—that may work best with AI/AN geroclients? Zitzow and Estes (1981, p. 138) recommended the following:

1. Reconsider the 50-minute hour; it may not always work.
2. Use the extended family to strengthen the dysfunctional one.
3. Don't press client in initial sessions.
4. Keep a low profile.
5. Keep confrontation, considered rude, to a minimum.
6. Respect AI/AN values but respond to client as a person first.

In planning interventions and arranging counseling sessions, group meetings, health clinic days, etc., it is necessary to learn about and consider the times, durations, and meanings of Indian feast days, healing ceremonies, mourning periods, celebrations, and social days. Know about traditional healing beliefs and about practices regarding fasting, food restrictions, sweat lodges, and use of herbs, and how they might affect prescriptions. Medications like insulin, for example, may have to be adjusted to ceremonies that involve changes in diet and activity. McCabe and Cuellar (1994) wrote that certain objects or skin marks on elders may be noted after healing ceremonies. You are advised to learn about them so as not to cite them as evidence of elder abuse.

Elder Abuse

Maxwell and Maxwell (1992) applied the social exchange theory of power to explain elder abuse in Indian tribes. This includes physical abuse like battering, primary neglect like consciously taking an elder's money or leaving a vulnerable elder alone for an extended time, and secondary neglect like neglecting a frail elder because of circumstances beyond the family member's control (excessive distance or job demands). Usually, one works with the family (not against it) in nonjudgmental ways to break the bonds of excessive two-way dependencies. Such problems are seen either as forms of psychopathology or as weakness of character, and consequences have ranged from therapy to imprisonment (or both). But always, the goal is cessation of the abuse.

According to these authors, the reason for treatment failures—as indicated by high recidivism in abuse and by continued substance abuse and mistreatment—is that interventions have focused only on individual traumas, not on collective trauma. It is easier to identify an individual as the locus of deviance, and we are less familiar with community-level approaches to aberrant behavior. Since one form of abuse leads to another, programs should address the structural antecedents (outer systems) of the social problems being treated, such as poverty, unemployment, apathy, and hopelessness.

It was also suggested that elders who live great distances from support systems be voluntarily "moved in" to senior centers for the winter months, an intervention which may not seem unreasonable to people with a nomadic heritage.

Alcoholism and Suicide

It would seem that the same systemic approaches would apply to the prevention and treatment of both alcoholism and suicide. Problems must be addressed at both the individual pole and the societal pole of the continuum. May (1985) called for creative and innovative interventions with the social and physical environment; legalization of alcohol in reservations where prohibition still exists; educational programs dealing with early developmental problems that might lead to misuse; and an upgrading of AI/AN rehabilitation programs through increased use of traditional tribal strengths and modern treatment modalities. Mail and Wright's (1989) article, "Point of View: Indian Sobriety Must Come from Indian Solutions," provides some directions.

Long-Term Care

On the Navajo reservation, a home health care project using life themes of elders from remote areas included:

1. Providers who spoke the Navajo language.
2. A base of traditional values such as responsibility for older persons and the importance of female kinship.
3. An understanding of the reluctance of grown children to make placement decisions for parents.
4. A respect for traditional beliefs about health and illness, such

as the link between health and correct relationships of person, environment, world, and others.

5. The use of diviners to diagnose and singers to heal. (Boyle, Syzmanski, & Syzmanski, 1992, p. 11)

The lack of Indian nursing homes and the prevalence of chronicity do not necessarily imply that nursing homes should be expanded. To the AI/AN, a nursing home may be a bad omen— a place to die—and therefore it may have a detrimental effect on the person's health. A nursing home out of range of tribal contacts or outside of a sacred region may also create adverse outcomes. In general, nursing homes that are owned and operated by a tribe, are located on the reservation, are staffed by both medicine persons and public health physicians, and offer Indian food and traditional activities appear to work out best.

Barriers

The continuum of long-term care on reservations is plagued by enormous distances and lack of transportation. Many eligible people do not receive care or information, so little can be done about promoting health, preventing sensory deprivation, controlling hypertension, etc. More creative outreach approaches (such as mobile clinics and voluntary winter relocations) are needed

Because the self-esteem of AI/ANs is strengthened through ethnicity and group identity, optimum medical and mental health services should revolve around natural neighborhoods (family and clan helping systems), and mental health programs should offer services based on ethnicity, differential environments, and extended family units.

Terminations in Ethnogerocounseling

There are many cultural norms to consider in family counseling with regard to end-of-life issues, and some may appear contradictory. For example, because AI/ANs have a circular time orientation, talking about death may be relatively easy; but Navajos believe that discussing death precipitates death and should be avoided. Decisions about long-term care may not fit into an AI/AN present-day orientation. Although the interdependent group is important, individual autonomy is even more highly valued, and the group will support the individual decision no matter how long it takes to be made. However, with an extended family or group orientation when an elder is incompetent, specifying a health care proxy may not be so difficult. Such a person is often designated in the elder's tribal code, or one will emerge informally.

An informal survey of providers of health care to American Indians found the following:

> Respondents agreed with the sense of the literature that autonomy is a very strongly held value among Indian people and that the family and group around a person would act as an advocate for that autonomy. Children would be very unlikely to interpose their interests or wishes in the matters of the kinds of end of life decisions a parent should make (Hepburn & Reed, 1995, p. 105)

These decisions usually emerge from roundabout, indirect conversations, such as talking about someone else in the community with the same problem; and it is not always clear to an outsider when a decision has been reached. Here, Hepburn and Reed suggested using a cultural, not necessarily a linguistic, interpreter. Obtaining a signed form of consent may evoke hostility, so it is important to translate such a form positively, in terms of the client's own desires and specifications. The usual structured approach to advance directives may involve too much detail for an AI/AN family that has already made a decision such as "no extraordinary lifesaving measures." If so, the patient and the family may become upset or even hopeless. In sum, these authors concluded with the following guidelines:

1. Use the elder's cultural orientation.
2. Use the family's communication style.
3. Use cultural interpreters.
4. Use the elder's family or group in its own shape and form.
5. Use spiritual as well as physical aids.

When death occurs, we know that a strong support system is beneficial to the bereaved, and urban Indians and others away from traditional cultures may feel especially isolated. One temptation might be to jump in and organize their bereavement; but recognizing that AI/ANs value self-reliance, AARP (1990) warned that it is wise to lend support, not lead. A few of AARP's suggestions may run counter to your usual way of working in the dominant culture:

1. If the bereaved becomes emotional in talking about death, refocus to tasks that need to be done.
2. Give time for consideration about what has to be done.
3. Back off if the person is reluctant to be personal.
4. Don't confront denial or push "good grieving" practices.
5. Don't extend physical comforts (hugs, pats, touches), but do use a gentle (not firm) handshake,
6. Don't sit too close; listen carefully to each client; don't speak for anyone; practice noninterference.
7. Learn the dying, death, and burial norms of each client.

Like most others, American Indians have modified many of their end-of-life customs. Traditional Dakotahs (Sioux) used to mourn by wailing loudly and gashing themselves with knives—to show their grief and also to protect the tribe from spirits retaliating for improper mourning. They conducted two burials: burial in the sky and earth burial.

After a deceased Dakotah's face was painted and the body was attired in finery, locks of hair were clipped for survivors and the body was sewn into an animal skin or blanket for protection from the elements. Then it was placed in a tree or a six-foot platform along with necessary provisions (food, clothing, specific identifying possessions). In the four days it took for the soul to travel from the living, the family observed a respectful reticence. The tribe presented gifts to the deceased, and then the body was buried in an earthen mound on a hill near the platform.

Today . . . Dakotahs practicing traditional ways still hold a ceremony marking the end of the mourning period. The grave is covered with a blanket or quilt, and either cloth for making new clothes or newly made clothes are presented. These possessions are later given to a tribe member. A dinner is often held in the tribal hall during which food and money are given away, and tribe members give speeches and sing songs. For Dakotahs practicing traditional way, performing these rites of passage is considered, as in ancient times, the only proper way to mourn a loved one. (AARP, 1990, p. 21)

Not all AI/ANs view or mourn death in the same way, but many believe that some form of grieving strengthens one's harmony with nature and other human beings.

Even though Cherokees believed the dead spirit ascended to a higher state of unconditional love and remained near to comfort survivors, they still grieved over the loss of the relationship and the person's physical presence. Navajos saw death as the end of all that was positive about the soul's experience, and they respected and feared contact with the dead. Like the Dakotahs, they believed that observing certain grieving rituals protected them from retaliation by a dead spirit.

A Navajo counselor, in discussing how non-Indian providers could work effectively with AI/ANs, said it would help for all to know about traditional mourning practices. Using her language, her advice is summarized below.

Navajos believe that the spirit stays in the body for 4 days after death to allow time for the family to say good-bye and observe proper mourning. During this time, family members do not shower (that would wash the spirit away), eat red meat, touch fire, dig in the ground, wear jewelry, or indulge in luxuries. Children—considered too tender and precious to be exposed to death—are kept away. Friends may come to offer support and condolences.

After the 4 days of mourning, the body must not be touched. Touching a corpse will adversely affect one's mental, physical, spiritual, emotional well-being. The body must now be buried immediately, usually in a simple casket. (If the burial does not take place in 4 days, the spirit will always be around and may take you or your loved ones.) Friends may be invited for lunch after the burial, but the purpose is simply to feed those who have come from a distance, the mood is never celebratory.

On the morning of the fifth day, the family digs up a yucca plant and the root is shaved down to the white yucca, to be used as soap. Family members wash their hair, faces, and arms with the yucca soap. Then, because the spirit, which is death, is no longer with them, it is okay to take a shower. Now they are purified, but mourning may continue—this depends on the individual.

Because death is respected, talking about it is taboo—until it happens. Mortuaries and objects previously associated with death are avoided. Most people die in hospitals.

Sometimes a person becomes imbalanced (depressed) during the mourning period and consults a medicine man, who may prescribe a ceremony in which he will sing chants. The depressed person will sing along with him and be washed with herbs. This ceremony can last from 1 to 9 days. Different ceremonies are used at different seasons (for example, in the springtime the ceremony focuses on rebirth). Meditation (thinking positive thoughts) is also used: "Holy people make us holy."

It is estimated that only 2.27 percent of AI/ANs—usually those on reservations—still observe traditional bereavement customs, but many symbols and fragments of the traditions live on today in some bicultural forms.

We do not know everything that works and does not work in the gerocounseling of AI/AN elders, and we are still in the pioneering stage, pooling theories and techniques. Most of what we learn will come from the AI/AN elders themselves and from their ethnic providers, for they have been solving problems and healing themselves for centuries.

EXERCISE

Think about the four elders described at the beginning of Part II. On the basis of the ethno-gerontology principles discussed, how would you devise a care plan for each? What would you include? What would you need to know? How would you proceed? Include both micro and macro interventions.

References

American Association of Retired Persons (1990). *Health risks and preventive care among older American Indians and Alaskan natives*. Washington, DC: AARP.

American Association of Retired Persons (1995). *A portrait of older minorities*. Washington, DC: AAARP.

American Association of Retired Persons Minority Affairs (1990). *Customs of bereavement: A guide for providing cross-cultural assistance*. Washington, DC: AARP.

Bean, L. (1976). California Indian shamanism and folk curing. In

W. Hand (Ed.), *American folk medicine: A symposium*. Berkeley: University of California Press, pp. 109–113.

Blanchard, E. (1983). The growth and development of American Indian and Alaska Native Children. In G. Powell (Ed.), *The Psychosocial development of minority group children*. New York: Brunner/Mazel, pp. 110–130.

Boyle, J., Szymanski, M.T., & Szymanski, E. (1992). Improving home health care of the Navajo. *Nursing Connections, 5* (4), 3–13.

Burlingame, V. (1995). *Gerocounseling: Counseling elders and their families*. New York: Springer.

Carrese, J. & Rhodes, L. (1995). Western bioethics on the Navajo reservation: Benefit or harm? *Jama 274, 10,* 826–829.

Curley, L. (1982). Indian elders: A failure of aging policy. *Generations, 6* (3), 28, 52.

Davis, K. (1995, September 3). Ethnic cleansing didn't start in Bosnia. *New York Times Week in Review,* 1, 6.

Erikson, E. (1950). *Childhood and society*. New York: Norton.

Green, J. (1995). *Cultural awareness in the human services; A Multiethnic approach* (2nd ed.). Boston: Allyn and Bacon.

Greenhouse, A., & Dodson, B. (n.d.). Working with Native Americans: Problems and solutions. Reno: Nevada Geriatric Education Center.

Hepburn, K., & Reed, R. (1995). Ethical and clinical issues with Native-American elders. *Clinics in Geriatric Medicine 11* (1), 97–110.

Ho, M. (1987). *Family therapy with ethnic minorities*. Newbury Park, CA: Sage.

Indian Health Service. (1991). *Trends in Indian health*. U.S. Department of Health and Human Services, Public Health Service. Washington, DC: U.S. Government Printing Office.

Johnson, D. (1994, July 3). Economies come to life on Indian reservation. *New York Times National,* 1, 18, 19.

Johnson, F., Cook, E., Kelleher, M., Kentopp, E., & Manniein, E. (1986). Life satisfaction of the elderly American Indian. *International Journal of Nursing Studies, 23* (3), 265–273.

Kittler, P., & Sucher, K. (1989). *Food and culture in America*. New York: Van Nostrand and Reinhold.

Kramer, B. J. (1990). Urban American Indian aging. Paper presented at American Society on Aging meetings, San Francisco, CA.

Kramer, B. J. (1992). Cross-cultural medicine a decade later-Health and aging of urban American Indians. *Western Journal of Medicine, 157* (3), 281–285.

Levy, J., & Kunitz, S. (1987). A suicide prevention program for Hopi youth. *Social Science and Medicine, 25*, 931–940.

McCabe, M. & Cuellar, J. (1994). *Aging and health: American Indian/Alaska Native elders* (2nd ed.). Palo Alto, CA: Stanford Geriatric Education Center.

Mail, P., & Wright, L. (1989). Point of view: Indian sobriety must come from Indian solutions. *Health Education 20* (5), 19–25.

Manson, S., Beals, M., Dick, R., & Duclos, C. (1989). Risk factors for suicide among Indian adolescents at a boarding school. *Public Health Report, 104,* 609–614.

Manson, S. (1994, May 6). American Indian Elders. Keynote address at American Indian Aging Conference: Enhancing the Provision of Care-Strategies and Barriers, Wausau, WI. Sponsored by Wisconsin Geriatric Education Center.

Manson, S., Shore, J., & Bloom, J. (1985). The depressive experience in American Indian communities: A challenge for psychiatric theory and diagnosis. In A. Kleinman & Y. Good (Eds.), *Culture and depression.* Berkeley: University of California Press.

Markides, K., & Mindel, C. (1987). *Aging and ethnicity.* Beverly Hills, CA: Sage.

Maxwell, E., & Maxwell, R. (1992). Insults to the body civil: Mistreatment in two plains Indian tribes. *Journal of Cross-Cultural Gerontology 7,* 3–23.

May, Phillip. (1985). Alcohol and drug misuse prevention programs for American Indians: Needs and opportunities. *Journal of Studies on Alcohol 47* (3), 187–195.

Metz, S. (1991). The Native American family. *Interfaith Family Journal, 10* (1), 5–7.

Morinis, E. (1982). "Getting straight": Behavioral patterns in a skid row Indian community. *Urban Anthropology 11,* 193–214.

National Indian Council on Aging (1981). *American Indian elderly: A national profile.* Albuquerque, NM: Author.

Redhorse, J. (1980). American Indian elders: Needs and aspirations in institutional and home health care. In E. Stanford (Ed.), *Minority aging: Policy issues for the '80s* (pp. 61–68). San Diego: San Diego State University.

Strong, C. (1984). Stress and caring for elderly relatives: Interpretations and coping strategies in an American Indian and white sample. *Gerontologist, 24* (3), 251–256.

Stuart, P., & Rathbone-McCuan, E. (1988). Indian elderly in the United States. In E. Rathbone-McCuan & B. Havens (Eds.), *North American elders: United States and Canadian perspectives.* New York: Greenwood, 235–254.

Sue, D. W., & Sue, D. (1990). *Counseling the culturally different: Theory and practice* (2nd ed.). New York: Wiley.

Trimble, J., & LaFramboise, T. (1985). American Indians and the counseling process: Culture, adaptation, and style. In P. Pedersen (Ed.), *Handbook of cross-cultural counseling and therapy,* (127–134). Westport, CT: Greenwood Press.

U.S. Bureau of the Census (1990). Selected characteristics of the population 65 years and over. *Elders in the United States.* Washington, DC: U.S. Government Printing Office.

Weibel-Orlando, J. (1989). Elders and elderlies: Well-being in old age. *American Indian Cultural Reservation Journal, 13,* 75–84.

Weibel-Orlando, J. (1990). Grandparenting styles: Native American perspectives. In J. Sokolovsky (Ed.), *The cultural context of aging.* New York: Bergin and Garvey.

Westermeyer, J., & Peake, E. (1983). A ten-year follow-up of alcoholic Native Americans in Minnesota. *American Journal of Psychiatry, 140* (2), 189–194.

Wilson, U. (1983). Nursing care of American Indian patients. In M. Orque, B. Bloch, & L. Monroy (Eds.), *Ethnic nursing care: A multi-cultural approach,* 271–295. St. Louis, MO: Mosby.

Wise, F., & Miller, N. (1983). The mental health of American Indian children. In G. Powell (Ed.), *The psychosocial development of minority group children.* New York: Brunner/Mazel.

Yee, B. (1991). *Variations in aging: Older minorities.* Galveston: Texas Consortium of Geriatric Education Centers.

Zitzow, D., & Estes, G. (1981). The heritage consistency continuum in counseling Native American children. In Spring Conference on Contemporary American Issues (Ed.), *American Indian Issues in Higher Education,* pp. 133–139.

Acknowledgments for Part II

In addition to the Geriatric Education Centers at Stanford University in Palo Alto, California, and Marquette University in Milwaukee, Wisconsin for generously sharing hard-to-find current literature on ethnicity, aging, and American Indians and Alaska Natives, many individuals also helped in the preparation of this part of the book.

I wish to also thank the AI/AN health and social service providers and experts who took time out of their busy schedules to grant me interviews, who critiqued this section, or who presented materials at workshops that I attended.

From Wisconsin tribes, I thank Sandra Schuyler, RN, Director, Milwaukee Indian Community; Health Community, Donna Dominick at Milwaukee Indian Economic Development Agency; Noreen Smith, Tribe Elder Abuse Leader; Deanna Bauman, Oneida Health Center; Patsy Delgado, MA, at Milwaukee Interfaith; David Besaw and Sharon Coates at the Ella Bresaw CBRF; Mark Caskey at the Health Heart; Sonny Smart, PhD., UW-Stevens Point; Martine Mizwa, PhD, at Peter Christiansen Health Center, Lac du Flambeau; Kevin Culhane, MD, Menominee Tribal Clinic, Keshena, Wisconsin; and the Honorable Jacqueline D. Schellinger, Milwaukee Circuit Court.

California tribal people include Alfred Cross, MSW, Instructor, American Indian Studies; James Luna, MSW, Counselor, LaJolla Reservation; and Edmund Castillo, PhD, American Indian Studies at Sonoma State University. From Colorado: Spero Manson, PhD, University of Colorado Health Sciences Center, Denver. From Arizona tribes: Aurelia J. Nehaitewa, MSW, at the Hopi Guidance Center; Ruth Truhul at Cochina County Services; Evelyn Turner at Yavapai Apache Senior Center, and Deborah Bonally, MSW at the Navajo Nation Department of Aging. From New Mexico: Toby Chavez, LISW, Indian Health Service in Santa Fe.

Also: Billy Rogers, PhD, University of Oklahoma; and Wilma Mankiller, Cherokee Nation. From Texas: Thomas Wilson, MA, retired, Department of the Interior.

PART III

Hispanic-Latino American (H-L) Elders

As immigrants from Mexico arrived, they descended on friends or relatives, where often several families were already crowded together. The laws of hospitality were inviolable; no one was denied a roof and food during the first days, but after a while each person was to fend for himself. They streamed in from towns south of the border, looking for work, with nothing on their backs, a bundle over their shoulders, and the will to get ahead in the Promised land where, they had been told, money grew on trees and a clever man could become an impressario with his own Cadillac and a blonde on his arm. . . . They had no idea of the hardships of exile, how they would be abused by their employers and persecuted by authorities, how much effort it would take to reunite their family, to bring their children and old people, or how great would be the pain of telling their friends goodbye and of leaving their dead behind. Neither were they warned that they would quickly loose their traditions, or that recollections would corrode and leave them without memories. (Allende, 1993, p. 41)

The Historical Context

1500	Colonization of New Spain begins.
1600	Mexicans live in the southwest.
1608	Santa Fe founded.
1821	Mexico wins independence from Spain.
1846–1848	Mexican-American War.
1850–1899	Gold Rush in California and Texas. Ranching lures Mexicans to Arizona despite anti-Mexican laws and practices.
1861–1865	American Civil War.
1899	First Puerto Rican immigration wave.
1910	Second Mexican immigration wave.
1913	Mexican revolution.
1914–1918	World War I.
1920–1928	500,000 Mexicans come on permanent visas for "coyote" industry, railroads, and manufacturing. Barrio and border patrols develop.
1928–1942	500,000 repatriated to Mexico; others segregated.
1929–1937	Great Depression.
1930s	Dust bowls.
1939–1945	World War II. 350,000 Mexicans serve. Other H-Las also serve. Increased Mexican immigration for war industries. First bracero program; anti-Mexican media coverage.
1947	Operation Bootstrap begins in Puerto Rico. Mexican-American ex-GIs organize for civil rights; 273,000 new documented Mexican immigrants; illegals are raided.
1959	Communist revolution in Cuba.
1959–1961	First Cuban immigration wave.
1960	Chicano movement begins.
1961–1965	Second Cuban immigration wave.
1964–1965	Civil rights legislation passed.
1965	Older Americans Act passed; Immigration and Nationality Act, favoring families.
1965–1973	Third Cuban immigration wave.
1970	H-Las migrate to the midwest; 85 percent urban. Widespread deportation of undocumented persons.

1980	H-Ls' pride in arts, media, and language develops. Amnesty program; deportations continue.
1980–1983	Fourth Cuban immigration wave.
1990s	Anti-immigration sentiment resumes.
1998	California votes to discontinue bilingual education.

Case Examples

Antonio, a Working-Class Mexican-American With Medical Problems and Minimal Support

Antonio Gonzales, age 55, came from a rural area near Guadalajara with his wife and four children to work in the fields in southeast Wisconsin. Some winters he was hired for foundry work. His wife died after their grown children had moved to the city for jobs.

Mr. Gonzales's health deteriorated, perhaps because of his hard-working life. His back was painfully arthritic, his knees were shot, and his lungs were damaged by poisonous pesticides. Weakened from labored breathing, he developed heart problems. At 50, he spoke little English, had little income and no medical insurance, and did not know that he was eligible for any benefits.

He was referred to the United Migrant Opportunity Services, which helped him get a medical card and got him into treatment that included knee replacements and medications for COPD, heart disease, and depression. Because he could not live alone, a grand-daughter—Juanita Gonzales—took him in.

Juanita Gonzales, a single mother with three small children, was attending technical school and working full-time. She had no child support, and her grandfather's expenses strained her budget. Often she had to miss classes to take him to medical appointments. She became depressed and quit school altogether.

Felicia Marquez, an Upper-Class Cuban American With Depression and Moderate Support

Felicia Marquez, age 76, is the oldest of five children of rich Cuban entrepreneurs. After attending the university, she married. Her husband, Arnoldo, was a physician. They had three children. Their life in Cuba was affluent and happy until the Communist Revolution in 1959; they fled in 1962. Arnoldo Marquez set up practice in Miami, and they maintained an upper-class Cuban lifestyle, though their children became 'decubanized.'

Felicia Marquez's siblings had stayed in Cuba to care for her ailing father and to save the family business. Guilty about leaving, she worked for a family reunion in 1972. By then, however, her father, the business, and the money were gone. Instead of a happy reunion, the next 25 years brought dissension and blaming. Often, the most heated arguments were political.

Mrs. Marquez felt that she had failed her family and tried, literally, to work herself out of her suffering. Priding herself on being a good daughter, wife, mother, grandmother, and housekeeper— but most of all a good Catholic—she tripled her efforts in each area. She and her siblings competed over being the mother's caregiver.

In confession, she told her priest that she believed she was paying for her sins. (Perhaps a *santería god* was angry at her.) Her own well-being was unimportant. Nobody appreciated her, and her own children paid more attention to their children than to her. The priest recognized that Mrs. Marquez was depressed. She admitted she was not sleeping and had lost 25 pounds in the past 3 months. But she said she was not suicidal—suicide "was a sin." The priest suggested prayers, a novena, and the stations of the cross. When these helped only partially, he advised her to consult her physician. She refused. She felt ashamed, and she wanted help from family or not at all.

Elena Rodriguez, a Puerto Rican-American From an Impoverished Environment, With Depression and Minimal Support

Elena Rodriguez, age 64, the eldest of five, was born in San Juan in 1933 to poor parents who migrated to New York City when Elena was 3. They hoped for employment and a better life but did not find either. The father became disabled from polio. The mother, overwhelmed with family responsibilities, had serious episodes of depression that required hospitalization. Neighbors helped but mostly Elena, who dropped out of school in ninth grade, kept house and cared for her siblings. The family, on general relief, survived marginally in Brooklyn and never revisited Puerto Rico.

Later Elena was proud to assure her mother she was a good girl and virgin when she married a coworker, Carlos Rodrieguz. Soon afterword, Marita and Pepe were born. The family was fairly happy despite financial struggles. Mrs. Rodriguez counseled her two sisters—one on drugs the other, a runaway—she nursed her sickly mother, and raised her own children. She never saw her brothers.

Carlos Rodriguez, a strict father and possessive husband, was protective of his family, but on weekends he partied with friends, leaving Mrs. Rodriguez at home. In 1970, he was fatally shot in a drive-by shooting. His wife said that her devotion to Catholicism, which incorporated what she called spiritualism and *espiritistas,* helped her through. She believed in *fatalismo,* that "there was always a reason."

When her mother developed cancer, Mrs. Rodriguez gave her herbs from Brazil and the West Indies as well the doctor's medicine. She sang a song at "Mommi's" funeral, honoring her as a "saint," knowing she was now entering the gates of heaven and all was now perfect.

Mrs. Rodriguez was referred to a Puerto Rican agency—the Instituto—by a home care worker because she was not eating or sleeping well, cried often, and wanted to die. Now obese, and with hypertension, gallstones, and heart disease, she was homebound, alone in public housing. Her children seldom came to see her. This was due to conflict over Marita's sexual behaviors—an illegitimate baby and a series of live-in boyfriends—and Pepe's gang membership, with its culture of drugs and jail.

Mrs. Rodriguez made no secret of the fact that her children were causing her illness and unhappiness. She herself had done what her mother wanted and had always been there for her mother. Now, at her own hour of need, her children were not there for her. This was her worst disappointment.

Although she was a law-abiding person, Mrs. Rodriguez had many confrontations with the legal system over Pepe's problems. She also felt ashamed about trying to get Marita and the baby onto AFDC. Therefore, she viewed the referral to the Instituto with suspicion.

Carmen M., a Spanish-speaking worker with both *personalismo* and *dignidad,* was assigned to her case. Ms. M. engaged Mrs. Rodriguez in talk about their homeland and offered concrete help with home services. Mrs. Rodriguez asked her some personal questions. Lonely and abandoned, she liked talking about commonalities and she got Ms. M. to do practical things—help move this; get that out of the refrigerator. Because of the client's many needs, the worker's visits lengthened. "Mrs. Rodriguez has no one to talk to," Mrs. M. told her supervisor, but she knew that these long visits were causing her to work overtime and to neglect her other clients.

Ms. M. and her supervisor revised the care plan. Because of the good rapport, she had developed with Mrs. Rodriguez, Ms. M. was able to explain the new limits so that the client would not feel rejected. A Spanish-speaking telephone reassurance service was tried and a goal was to enlist Marita. Ms. M. advised Marita: "Even if you don't think your mother deserves your special attention now, you might feel better about yourself for helping her—so do it for yourself. It is *familismo*."

Ms. M knew that Mrs. Rodriguez would soon need a nursing home. The client was relying heavily on home remedies from botanicas and herbalists, and she liked spicy, salty foods; thus she was noncompliant with her medical regimen. Ms. M. was surprised when Pepe and Marita vetoed the nursing home, saying, "We don't believe in that." Ms. M. felt stuck.

Maria Martinez, Working-Class, From Santo Domingo With Dementia and Good Support; and Her Caregiver Daughter, Lily Rivas

Maria Martinez, age 80, from a rural area in the Dominican Republic, went through eighth grade and then did factory work until her marriage and the births of Lily and Emanuel. Soon after that, she divorced. She then cared for her parents. When they died, she migrated to New York City.

Obese since adolescence, Mrs. Martinez became an insulin-dependent diabetic. She was often noncompliant about diet, medication, and exercise, and she developed complications—neuropathy, kidney problems, and eye problems. At age 70, she experienced memory problems, which she attributed to "old age."

She moved in with her daughter Lily Rivas, Lily's daughter Rosalie, and Rosalie's two small children. But Mrs. Martinez complained about the noise, felt neglected, and refused to help out in this busy four-generation family. So when they learned of an opening in a senior apartment building where most residents were Spanish-speaking, all welcomed the move. Although Lily Rivas remained attentive, Mrs. Martinez's discontent continued. She visited her island several times, giving Lily a respite, but she was always worse when she returned. As her health and finances diminished, her trips ceased. Now Mrs. Rivas checked on her mother three times daily, in addition to holding a job and caring for the grandchildren. Consulting her physician, she admitted that she was hiding her burdens for fear that she would be labeled a "bad daughter"—or worse that her mother would be labeled a "crazy person." She also feared unaffordable expenses ahead. All this was her "cross to bear."

Mrs. Rivas was assured that Mrs. Martinez was eligible for home care and other services. Tests done at the Senior Assessment Center confirmed early-stage Alzheimer's disease, and a dementia day program at the Spanish-speaking Community Caregiving Program was recommended. Also, Mrs. Rivas was encouraged to attend the caregivers' support group and to do some reading about the disease, to understand that her mother was not "crazy."

But Mrs. Martinez refused to consider the day center. She felt that it was "the daughter's place" to care for the mother. The day care worker suggested not forcing her, but rather bringing her there as an "outing." Once Mrs. Martinez was there, she forgot her refusal to attend and wanted to stay all day. She called the group activities "the show."

Mrs. Martinez now enjoys her daily group of peers, the lunch, the show, and singing songs she had forgotten. While her memory worsens and her chronic poor health continues, she has an improved quality of life and complains less. The day care worker instills the idea that "we are born to have fun," believing that dementia victims can enjoy life and develop. She sees more progress than the family, because they compare her present condition with the past. "Here," the worker says, "we know them only as they are now and as they were when they came to us."

Mrs. Rivas's life has improved too. At 59, she is still a conscientious caregiver, running errands and showing love—but now with less resentment and guilt, knowing her burden is shared. Mrs. Martinez, diagnosed with Alzheimer's disease with concurrent hypertension, has been able to stay out of a nursing home through assisted living—although Lily Rivas accepts the eventual possibility of a nursing home. Staff members are paving the way by suggesting she take one day at a time and when the need arises, they will help with plans and adjustments.

While she strives to make her Spanish-speaking group culturally specific, the leader also sees dementia as a leveler that wipes away the boundaries of class, race, and ethnicity. It is a state in which clients connect on a human but preverbal level, she said.

Juan Perez, a Working-Class Mexican-American With Dementia and Strong Support; and Alicia Perez, His Caregiver

Juan and Alicia Perez, both in their mid-sixties, immigrated in 1942 to work in the war industry but ended up in a canning factory in Salinas, California. They raised six children, now married and living around Los Angeles. Five years ago, Juan, who had been acting "confused and forgetful" for some time, was informally diagnosed with Alzheimer's disease. As he was still ineligible for Medicare, Alicia Perez worked to pay for health insurance.

The Perez's oldest daughter, Dolores Segura, came weekly to help. She and Alicia Perez covertly competed over who was the boss or caretaker, but Mrs. Segura never openly disagreed, even when her mother was wrong. She believed her mother was doing too much, was too rigid, had become a martyr, needed to get out, and should start considering a nursing home. She was afraid that her mother too would become ill and she discussed this with Maria L., a worker at the office of the Alzheimer's Association.

Ms. L. knew what Alicia Perez needed—more information, more support, and more respite—but she also knew the culture of Mexican-American women in Salinas. She expected resistance to her initial outreach, and so she planned wisely. First (in Spanish) she offered concrete help, setting up a free dementia assessment at Stanford. Important information about the disease and caregiving followed. Next she suggested a day care center for Mr. Perez while Mrs. Perez attended a support group. But Mrs. Perez said no, giving numerous excuses—her homemaking schedule was inflexible; supper started in the afternoon and was served at five; then she had to clean up and get Mr. Perez to bed. She had to do it all.

Ms. L. said that the group meetings did not start until late and pointed out that this wasn't a group where you had to say bad things about your loved one but simply a group where you learned to be a better caregiver. It would be a party with food and music. She would call to remind Mrs. Perez the night before. Finally, Mrs. Perez agreed. She soon enjoyed coming—and bringing and sharing food. Later, the group (which consisted of about 10 families) agreed to join a more formal study group. The members were even paid for their participation and transported in a van. "It was the first Spanish-speaking group on wheels," Ms. L. said.

Now, after 5 years, the group meets informally on its own. The members no longer hide the "shame of Alzheimer's" but invite public speakers to give up-to-date information on dementia. They call themselves the *Grupo de Apoyo*—a change, Ms. L. said, from "I don't need help" to "help is okay." Juan Perez goes to day care three times a week, and Alicia Perez feels supported and able to keep him home.

Carlos Hernandos, a Working-Class Mexican-American With Alcoholism and Moderate Support

Every June for 5 years, Carlos Hernandos, now 59, and his three sons came to Kenosha, Wisconsin, to pick cabbages. They returned to Laredo, Texas, each October. During these summers, Mr. Hernandos missed his wife. When he was hired for a year-round factory job in Kenosha, the family moved.

Mr. Hernandos began drinking in his teens. Like many of his *compadres* and even many of his relatives, he believed that after a hard day's work in the sun, alcohol was a just reward. Eventually he was up to a six-pack daily; then he added tequila, and then pot. When he was drunk, he slept in the backyard on a cot so as not to disturb the family.

In 1996, Mr. Hernandos was arrested for driving while intoxicated. He was then hospitalized for detox. In the hospital, he was told that he had cirrhosis of the liver. Alcohol counseling had been ordered by the court, but he refused inpatient treatment because he had to support his family. The counseling fared no better. Mark T., his counselor, was a white man who struck him as phony and uninterested.

Mr. Hernandos did not consider himself an alcoholic; nor did he see drinking as a disease connected to his ill health. The only thing wrong with his drinking, he felt, was that it had caused an arrest and a fine. He was ashamed of getting caught. He hated the AA meetings where he had to say he would always be an "alcoholic" and must quit drinking altogether. He wouldn't go along with that.

But priding himself on being a smart person, he agreed with his counselor, to fulfill the court's requirement and get it over with. He promised himself secretly that next time he would find a nondrinking, designated driver or walk home and not get into such a mess again. After the required sessions, Mark T. closed the case.

Chapter 7

The H-L Ethnic Lens

Now, let us look through the H-L ethnic lens, with a special emphasis on Mexican, Puerto Rican, and Cuban American elders and their families. As we do, think of the fictional case examples at the beginning of this section and also refer to the historical context.

Identity

In 1978, the United States government formally defined the Hispanic ethnic category as including people of Mexican, Puerto Rican, Cuban, Central or South American, or other Spanish cultures or origins, regardless of race. Because this classification can be confusing, terms specifying national origins, historical time frames, languages, racial ascriptions, religious affiliations, political leanings, surnames, individual preferences, and other forms of cultural identification and custom are also used.

While these modifiers help to establish an identity among a people, we must consider the Hispanic-Latino/a (H-L) lens as a complex category comprising many diverse cultures, each with its own variables interacting with the social structures of the others and the dominant culture in a systemic process. Our focus will often be at an interface.

Gonzalez (1991) proposed the term Hispanic/Latino, reasoning that Hispanic has been the usage of the last two decades and Latino (preferred by most Spanish-speaking peoples) will be that of the future. AARP (1990) pointed out that Hispanic is preferred on the East Coast by Puerto Ricans and Cubans, but Latino and Chicano are preferred on the West and by younger people.

Identity also defines political status. H-Ls are native-born, naturalized citizens; temporary migrant workers; or documented or undocumented refugees—all from Latin America. The refugees often pejoratively labeled "legals" or "illegals," continue to be a subject of controversy in the United States. Chicano, La Raza, and Mestizo are also used.

The importance of categories extends beyond political correctness. A serious problem in research is that it is often unclear who constitutes the H-Ls under study. Some analysts use subgroups; others do not, making it difficult to generalize. Here, we will use Hispanic-Latino (H-L) officially and also Spanish-speaking, Mexican, Puerto Rican, and Cuban American when applicable.

H-L racial origins also vary. The 1990 U.S. Census removed Hispanics from the race category after 11.5 million identified themselves as white, 77,000 as black, 165,000 as American Indian, 305,000 as Asian, and 915 million as "other." Societies, Montalvo (1991) wrote, classify individuals as being racially alike or different on the basis of phenotypes (skin color, physiognomic features, etc.). H-L phenotypes are:

1. *Blancas,* a light group of whites born in Latin America, who are considered elite.
2. *Mestizos,* Mexicans of Indian and Iberian roots, who range from the light *trigeños* (the color of wheat) to *mulattoes* (the Afro-Iberians) and who comprise some 30 separate groups formed from such mixtures, each with a different social standing.
3. *Dark people,* Indios and Negroes, who suffer the most discrimination.

Racial characteristics were important in Latin American life during the Spanish colonial period because they affected rights, privileges, and responsibilities. Mexico's complex caste system was abolished in 1821, at the time of the Spanish-Mexican War of

Independence. Still, three major social or color groups persist—the light, intermediate, and dark phenotypes—and the message has been, "The whiter the better."

Puerto Ricans are more tolerant and accepting of color differences, even within the same family. Silva (personal communication, 1995) attributed this to their past history, when they were almost "wiped out." Ragau (personal communication, 1997) said that she thought there was color prejudice; her Puerto Rican father would say, "Bottom-line, look at my skin." Before Castro's regime, Cubans had a color caste system, with whites at the top; but after the revolution, whites became suspect as sympathizers with the United States.

Demographics

Accurate data on this population are hard to come by. The 1990 Census counted 21 million people of Spanish origin, making up 8 percent of the total U.S. population. This was a 40 percent increase from 1980. A 200 percent increase is predicted from 1990 to 2008. At current rates, H-Ls will be the largest minority by 2020, totaling 15 percent of the U.S. population (AARP, 1995).

H-Ls are a very young population; their average age is 26, 9 years younger than non-H-Ls. In 1990, 1.2 million (5 percent) of the 21 million Hispanics were over 65 and 94,000 (1 percent) were over 85 years; these two were the fastest-growing age groups among H-Ls. There are 100 older women for every 71 older men. As with white elders, twice as many men as women over 65 are married and living with a spouse (AARP Minority Affairs, 1995).

Most older H-Ls live in four states; Mexicans and Central Americans tend to live in California and Texas, Cubans in Florida, Puerto Ricans and Caribbeans in New York.

H-L elders mostly remain in the community. Only 2.7 percent were in institutions in 1985, compared with 7.8 percent blacks (AARP Minority Affairs, 1995). Three-fourths (76.6 percent) lived in mostly multigenerational households, and 22 percent lived alone (U.S. Bureau of the Census, 1991). H-L elders are less likely than other elders to own a car or a home; most still live in *barrios*, Spanish enclaves that served as buffers against the outside world but now are crime-ridden. Safe, affordable housing and accessible transportation to health and social services are urgently needed.

The 1990 median per capita income for all older Hispanics was slightly above the poverty line—for females, $5,543; for males, $8,486—and 22.5 percent are below the poverty level (compared with 10 percent of whites). Poverty is highest among women and nonmetropolitan elders (AARP, Minority Affairs, 1995).

Older H-Ls are less likely than whites to receive Social Security. If they do receive it, they are more likely to receive minimum benefits because of lower-paying prior employment. Twenty-one percent received Supplemental Security Income (SSI), compared with 7 percent of all other elders. It is estimated that H-L elders are more likely to be unemployed than those in other categories. Cuban elders, who tend to have earned higher wages, are most likely to be employed; Puerto Ricans are more likely to be employed than Mexicans. Puerto Ricans and Mexicans have reported low lifetime wages and being physically unable to work in old age (Villa, Cuellar, Gamel, & Yeo, 1993).

H-L immigration has differed from that of other ethnic categories. Asians and Europeans, seeking a better life, immigrated unilaterally in movements with clear historical demarcations. H-Ls moved bilaterally, and their immigration has often resembled a revolving door. Many arrived and left because of pull-push events in the United States; that is, a demand for cheap labor periodically pulled them here, but then they were pushed out when the economy no longer needed them. But family ties also pulled them back home—unlike Asian Americans, who were too far away from their homes to go back. As a result, most Asian Americans acculturated by the third generation whereas most H-Ls did not. The revolving-door effect has also made it difficult to provide services to H-Ls.

H-L immigrations occurred in different ways, and so we must know about each major subcategory.

Mexican Americans inhabited the U.S. Southwest before 1600 and before any Anglo settlements. After the Mexican-American War (1846–1848), Spain ceded this region to the United States, and their descendants became U.S. citizens.

The second mass entry consisted of over 1 million Mexicans escaping the violence of the Mexican Revolution of 1910, lured by promises of safety and employment in menial agricultural, industrial, and railroad jobs. Their numbers grew steadily until the Great Depression, when thousands were deported. This was in keeping with a prevailing prejudice against nonwhite immigrants, though as between Mexicans and Asians, Mexicans were seen as the lesser of two evils.

The Immigration Reform and Control Act of 1965 eased immigration quotas and reunified immigrant families, but some anti-Mexican feeling persists, as seen in 1994, in California's Proposition 187.

Puerto Rican Americans migrated in three major waves. The first (1899–1940) occurred after the United States invaded Puerto Rico in the Spanish-American War. Forced to find work, over 90,000 uneducated, unskilled, landless peasants, like Mrs. Rodriguez's parents, migrated to the mainland, where they found low-wage jobs or remained unemployed.

The second wave occurred after World War II, when capitalists on the mainland were offered long-term tax incentives to develop the Puerto Rican economy. This strategy, Operation Bootstrap (1947), also led to a massive migration of excess workers to the United States—and to the sterilization of low-income women, sometimes involuntarily, for "family planning" (Maldono-Dennis, 1969). By 1969, 35 percent of Puerto Rican women age 20–49 (today's younger elders), had been sterilized (Facundo, 1991). Although huge pharmaceutical plants were built on the island, migration continued in a third wave, resulting in a massive exodus of 2.5 million Puerto Ricans (12.7 percent of all H-Ls) by 1988.

Operation Bootstrap created two diverse groups—those who came and those who stayed—and their different beliefs and lifestyles make it impossible to lump Puerto Ricans together. A third group—health and social service workers—is currently being recruited so that providers and clients will share the same culture; but because of vast socioeconomic differences, this has not always worked (Comas-Diaz and Griffith, 1987).

Cuban Americans, numbering 1 million (10 percent of the island's population), immigrated to the United States in four waves after the Communist Revolution of 1959. Unlike other H-Ls, these Cubans tended to be affluent and well-educated, and to achieve financial, political, and professional success in the United States. The first wave (1959–1961) consisted of voluntary immigrants who did not plan to stay for more than a year but had to alter their plans after the failed invasion of the Bay of Pigs. Hernandez (1992) wrote that this group never accepted its status as an ethnic minority, and its members are sometimes called the "real refugees."

Those in the second Cuban wave (1961–1965) came later expecting more permanency. The third wave (1965–1973) arrived when U.S. Freedom Flights attempted to unite Cuban families. This Family Unification Program brought in middle-class skilled laborers, women, and white Cubans. Families were united, but like Felicia Marquez's family, they often had negative feelings about their previous separation (Hernandez, 1992).

Cuba's fourth wave (1980 and after) was precipitated by an incident at the Peruvian Embassy in Havana that resulted in the immigration of over 125,000 Cubans, mostly Marielitos (people who do not share the values of the Cuban dominant culture).

Cultural Values

There is no single H-L culture. H-Ls have many differences between and within socioeconomic, geographical, racial, and linguistic categories. These differences affect loyalties, political histories, local customs, and immigration or migration experiences.

H-Ls come from more than 26 nations. While most are Spanish-speaking (some using regional dialects), 3.05 percent who are not Spanish use other major European languages or English; but 39.3 percent of Mexican and Puerto Rican American elders have reported that they speak no English at all. Many H-Ls speak American Indian languages, creole dialects, and "Spanglish." Not all of the Spanish-speakers are fluent or literate in Spanish.

Roman Catholicism is their major religion, but Protestantism is growing. Some sects are influenced by African and Native American belief systems that have created their own forms.

Curanderismo—a holistic philosophy—is important, evidently permeating H-L culture, though there is considerable disagreement about its prevalence. Some researchers have found little evidence of practicing *cuaranderos,* or faith healers, today (Marquez, personal communication, 1995; Villa et. al., 1993); others describe it as a coherent worldview still held by many H-L elders (Valverde, personal communication, 1995; Yaniz, personal communication, 1995; Maduro, 1983). A folk philosophy and a healing system, *curanderismo* includes culturally-patterned beliefs about life, health, illness, and care. Here are some examples:

1. Disease, illness, and trouble come from strong emotional states or a lack of balance or harmony with one's environment (*expiritismo*).
2. Often a person is an innocent victim of evil forces (*espiritismo*).
3. Soul and body are one, but loss of soul is possible (*espiritismo*).
4. The natural and supernatural worlds are almost one (*espiritismo*).
5. Interdependence in a family requires family interventions in problems (*familismo*).
6. Relationships should be structured and respected according to a hierarchy (*familismo y jeraquismo*).
7. Illness can bring secondary gains to the family and to society (*familismo*).
8. Value is given to the present time (*presentismo*).

Knowing about these traditional values can help make you culturally sensitive whether your H-L geroclient embraces or rejects them.

Food is also important. In Mexico, the diet of 40 percent of the population falls below the minimum dietary standards set by the World Health Organization (WHO); and very high rates of malnutrition and obesity are seen in the United States, too. Being overweight is sometimes considered normal, and a symbol of health and well-being, for married women.

Some H-Ls, like some Asians, have a "hot-cold" theory about health and diet, believing that since the world's resources are limited, we must stay in harmony and balance with the environment. Methods of food preparation and effects of food on the body are said to be related to proximity to the sun. Hot connotes strength, and cold connotes weakness. Illnesses are either "hot" or "cold," and the opposite kind of food would be used for treatment.

A combination of traditional methods (a unique blend of Indian and Spanish, with corn, beans, tortillas, and chilies as staples) and American methods are seen in Mexican kitchens. Beer and tequila are enjoyed.

Native Puerto Rican foods are a blend of Spanish and indigenous offerings such as fruits (plantain, jobo, guanabana, star apples) and seafood, often flavored with ginger, oregano, and cilantro. Rice and black beans are staples.

Cubans blend Spanish and African traditions with island fruits and vegetables. Rice and cornmeal are staples, and arroz con pollo and picadillo are favorite stews. Good rum, coffee, and cigars add zest.

Because many newer immigrants are unfamiliar with modern cooking conveniences, they usually fry and grill rather than bake or boil and they avoid unfamiliar canned and frozen foods. More acculturated immigrants tend to use many prepared convenience foods and to like extra meat. They usually adapt their traditional eating patterns in the United States. According to one study, when they are given a choice in hospitals and nursing homes, they prefer to eat as Americans ate about 10 years ago (Kittler & Sucher, 1989).

Issues: Sources of Pain and Pride

Are H-Ls victims of their culture? Or is that idea a form of blaming the victim in order to absolve the mainstream? If the host country's goal was to put H-L immigrants into a "melting pot" and make them monolingual and monocultural, it has seldom worked. When it has worked, wrote Buriel (1984), that has been to the disadvantage of both sides. H-L young people who held to the traditional culture, such as language, made better academic and economic progress here and were less likely to fall into deviance. Efforts to bring about rapid acculturation only increased anxiety and stress; Mexican Americans who became bicultural too rapidly seem to have experienced the most psychosocial dysfunction. Buriel cited some second-generation males who chose escapist and alcohol-related behaviors as a means of coping with cultural conflicts.

H-Ls have high rates of poverty, unemployment, crime, drug abuse, gang activity, and teenage pregnancy. Many elders who worked hard and sacrificed much to provide their families with better lives are disappointed that their dreams did not come true and that acculturation appears to compound intergenerational stress.

Racism and discrimination against H-Ls persists in the United States today. Despite U.S. citizenship, H-Ls often continue to be treated as foreigners. Lately, many Americans, including some H-Ls themselves, stereotype the new immigrants as uneducated, unskilled, and unmotivated—future welfare recipients—and express concern about the large number of H-L immigrants.

One *cuaranderismo* belief is that difficulties can also bring benefits. An example may be in California's Proposition 187, which tried to cut off benefits but actually motivated thousands of undocumented H-Ls to apply for citizenship and to seek political empowerment. Other negative trends have also strengthened group and cultural identity. To H-Ls, "acculturation stress" is considered an ethnic phenomenon to which Anglos are immune. When an H-L accepts that belief, cultural identification with La Raza is reinforced (Keefe & Padilla, 1987). This way of thinking is not a panacea, and it is perhaps not always desirable, but it is a way of turning lemons into lemonade.

Strengths: Sources of Pride

The strengths and contributions of H-Ls are many. So much has been written about the problems of these proud peoples that their contributions are often overlooked. Despite a long history of discrimination in the United States, H-Ls have risked their lives to fight bravely in the nation's causes. Some—such as Edward R. Roybal, Blandina Cardeñas, Katherine Davalos Ortega, Fernando Torres-Gil, Luis Nogales, Federico Peña, Matt Rodriguez, and Illeana Ros-Lehtinen—served in top government positions.

H-L Americans have excelled in law, education, medicine, labor unions, and politics. They have advanced civil rights for minorities and the working poor. Examples include Caesar Chavez, Reis Lopez Tijerina, William Velasquez, Blandina Cardeñas Ramirez, Patrick Flores, Antonio Novello, Dolores Huerta, Velma Martinez, and Father Felix Varela.

Combining United States culture with Mayan, Aztec, Colonial Spanish, or African, many—such as Ferdinand Cestero, Osiris Delgado, Abelardo Diaz Alfaro, Jose de Diego, Juan Ramon Jimenez, Francisco Oller y Cesteros, and Lourdes Lopez—made contributions to the arts internationally.

Gloria Estefan, Andy Garcia, Paul Rodriguez, Jose Feliciano, Edward James Olmos, Jose Ferrer, Raul Julia, Rene Marques, and Rita Moreno have succeeded in entertainment. In education, there are Vilma Martinez, Jaime Escalante, and others; in business, Luis

Nogales, Roberto C. Goizueeta, Carolina Herrera, and many more. The list of top athletes includes Felipe Alou, Gigi Fernandez, Nancy Lopez, Orlando Cepeda, and Roberto Clemente. Ellen Ochoa is an astronaut.

And many more H-Ls—too numerous to mention—have contributed to bettering the United States and the world. Your H-L elder clients are proud of these people. As will be seen in Chapter 8, H-Ls often have especially admirable qualities: a loving nature, a loyal dedication to family values, and a firm work ethic.

EXERCISE

Think about our H-L case studies and any other H-L elders you may know. How could any of the historical events listed at the beginning of this chapter have affected their lives, their current problems, or the problems of their cohort? Consider the dimensions of the Ethnic Lens: identity, demographics, immigration and migration experiences, cultural values, and special issues. What part might any of these play in their present problems, beliefs, and attitudes? How will they affect your work?

Chapter 8

The H-L Gero Chi Lens

Now let us place the H-L lens on the Geo Chi Model, for additional insights. Again, you are warned not to overgeneralize about ethnic peoples; there are countless variations on each ethnic theme. This chapter will focus mainly on traditional H-L elders interacting with other family members who may be of different generations and at different levels of acculturation. Because these differences can create family tensions as well as growth, you need to know about each cohort.

The Ethnic Lens affects themes that have endured over time and includes attitudes and prescriptions about the biopsychosocial aspects of life. As you read, think about the H-L case examples. How does each fit into the H-L Gero Chi Model?

The Self-System

The Anglo-American "self" tends to be individualistic and egocentric. By contrast, the H-L "self" tends to be family-centric, a self within a family. *Familismo* means that the family takes precedence over self-development, but it is not in conflict with *personalismo*, which implies respect for the uniqueness and fundamental worth of each person—not for one's achievements or assets but for oneself. *Personalisimo* is unconditional regard; it requires caring and respect for all.

Self-concept, the cognitive definition of one's identity—usually based on life roles and the expectations of others—is complex and can be damaged in aging, as roles recede, shift, are lost, or are not realized. This can be particularly true for the immigrant elder.

Self-esteem, the emotional evaluation of oneself, can also be at risk with H-Ls and other ethnic peoples because of years of discrimination due to race or gender (or both), in addition to losses experienced in immigration, acculturation, and aging.

Self-esteem is rooted in cultural values. In the dominant society, status is related to marketable skills, so there is a link between modernization and the lowered status of older persons. This is even more true for Hispanic elders, many of whom were socialized with agrarian values and expertise passed down to succeeding generations, in the expectation that their wisdom would be valued and that they would be supported in old age as a moral obligation. People turned to relatives for help first; a good old age relied on family support; self-esteem was based on the family.

But if the expertise of elders lost value through mobility, modernization, and acculturation, and if the family broke down, many elders became isolated, a burden, or simply unimportant. The result was lower self-esteem and a higher incidence of mental illness (Korte, 1978).

Because feeling "old" is often related to poor health, the inability to work, and feeling useless and unhappy, H-Ls, like American Indians, often consider themselves "old" as early as age 45. (Blacks, on average, report feeling "old" at 63, Anglos at about 70). H-Ls tend to be more pessimistic than other groups; over half of H-L elders in one study perceived old age as undesirable (Korte, 1978).

The self has many facets. In this model, we highlight two aspects of the self—gender and spirituality—because of their special significance in aging. They are influenced by and influence the other systems in the Gero Chi Lens.

Gender

Although the majority of H-L elders (58.4 percent) are female, this represents a gender gap narrower than that of blacks or whites; the reason is that H-L women have a shorter life expectancy. More older males (73 percent) than females (40 percent) are married.

Many H-L elder subgroups observe a tradition of *machismo* and *marianismo,* which provides highly structured gender prescriptions with nationalistic and religious roots. Unfortunately, such patterns have been misunderstood, unfairly judged in their extreme forms, and used as stereotypes to describe "a brutal, uncaring macho male" and a "masochistically suffering, depressed female" (Maduro, 1983, p. 872).

Maschismo comes from a patriarchal system of male authority and leadership. The male, protector of female and family, is supposed to be strong, providing, and in control; to live by a code of male honor; to represent the family in the community; to ensure family honor; and to regulate standards of respectability. A man with *machismo* has "honor, dignity, and pride, all expressed in the orderly hierarchical relationships of the household" (Green, 1995, p. 262). The macho ideal, wrote Maduro, "is not that of an authoritarian, belligerent, or insensitive man but, in a positive sense, an individualistic man with dignity who provides and cares for people with whom he is in close contact" (1983, p. 872).

In the United States, however, many elder males have experienced frustration because they lack language and job skills, because they are powerless after years of discrimination and poverty, and finally because they are weakened by premature, often work-related, physical problems. In many cases, the result is an isolated, depressed older male who feels impotent and expectations about his role—in terms of gender and age—are in conflict with the reality of life in the United States. Such conditions can make him defensive and tough with his family, or unable to work well with authorities or with the agencies trying to help him.

Marianismo, the Hispanic-Latina ideal, is symbolized by the Virgin Mary, the blessed mother. A "good woman" is restrained, submissive, spiritually sensitive, and self-sacrificing for husband and family; this is considered a most sacred, prestigious, and powerful role, to be exercised quietly. She is outwardly dependent and docile with men, yet a capable home manager. The H-L woman has proved to be accomplished when the man migrated, leaving her in charge.

Mixed messages about gender create conflicts and tensions for some H-L elder women and their daughters, and much has been written about the hypothesis that they are in "triple jeopardy"—being old, Hispanic, and female. Bastida and Jurez (1991) noted H-L older women:

1. Some researchers conclude that they are more depressed and unhappy than males; others have found no differences.
2. Some say they are more likely to live in multigenerational households; others find them more alone.
3. Some say they are dependent; others report that women are more resourceful but used different coping mechanisms, like manipulation, interpersonal skills, and the exchange of resources for services or support.
4. Older H-L women are poorer and sicker than males.

Silva (personal communication, 1995) said that the male-female balance was often disrupted by the economics of immigration. Some H-L females had superior fine motor skills as a result of years of needlework and thus were more marketable and better-paid than their husbands, whose work was agricultural. When women had higher salaries, divorce, although unacceptable to most, became possible if desired.

While some critics protest a system that encourages women to feel inferior and reinforces the role of martyr, others react differently. "These traditional sexual codes seem to condone the oppression of one group (female) by another (male) ... but relationships between the sexes are not straightforward (Comas-Diaz, 1987, p. 463). Allende (1993) wrote:

> The father's authority was never questioned: I wear the pants here, Pedro Morales roared whenever anyone trod on his toes, but in fact Inmaculada was the true head of the family. No one approached the father directly, [because everyone preferred] to be processed through the maternal bureaucracy. Inmaculada never contradicted her husband before witnesses but always managed somehow to get her way. (71–72)

Spirituality

Hispanic Christianity was influenced by Spanish, African, and American Indian belief systems. Most H-Ls are Roman Catholic—as has already been noted—but Protestantism is growing. While religion and spirituality are not necessarily the same, to most H-L elders, religion, spirituality, *curanderismo,* and healing practices can often be seen as one. Balance and harmony of life's emotional, physical, and social aspects are achieved by mixing, coming together, ritual fusion, and communion (Maduro, 1983). *Botanicas,* for example, are stores that sell herbal medicine and religious images and are also communal centers for the expression of the spiritist beliefs of *santeria* (Castez, 1994).

Mestizo-Roman Catholic ideas that influence H-L culture and personality development include these ideas:

1. Today's sacrifice brings tomorrow's salvation.
2. Being charitable to others is a virtue.
3. Endure wrongs against you (turn the other cheek).
4. Problems or events are meant to be.
5. Religion is the major resource; go to the priest for help.
6. Human nature, governed by supernatural forces, is a mixture of good and bad.
7. The person is naturally neutral and can be changed.

Curanderismo, introduced earlier, is a set of folk beliefs that permeates Hispanic spirituality. Strongly linked to religion, it is a form of self-actualization with aspects of positive healing. Its two major assumptions are (1) that the natural world is not clearly separate from the supernatural, and (2) that body and soul are one, but the living can experience loss of soul. Therefore propitiation, prayers, penance, miracles, vows—and any similar attempts to induce the gods and saints to grant requests (such as a request to regain the soul)—are common (Maduro, 1983). Even though Alicia Perez received much scientific information about her husband's Alzheimer's disease, she never let go of the belief that Juan's soul had been lost, and she daily prayed to the saints for a miracle.

To many H-Ls, the soul has a body, but a soul can be lost or can "travel in dreams." This has been likened to depersonalization or derealization in Western psychiatry. *Susto* (natural fright from physical, social, or emotional events) can create loss of soul and hence bodily ills. *Curanderos* and *curanderas* (folk healers) treat first the soul (psyche) and then (or not at all) the body. *Curanderismo* healing encompasses liberation, empowerment, guidance, and communion with God or some other higher power.

Espiritismo, a similar but more intellectual philosophical system with spiritual and religious components, is popular among Puerto

Ricans. Mrs. Rodriguez in the case history, believed that the dead could communicate with the living, and she often talked to her mother's spirit. Later, instead of seeing this as a form of schizophrenic hallucinating, Carmen—her case manager—used and reframed Mrs. Rodriguez's *espiritismo* by asking often, "What would your deceased mother advise you to do about this now?"

Santeria, a combination of religion and witchcraft, is primarily a Cuban-African system. Some Catholic saints' names reflect African beliefs such as *las siete potencias africanas. Santeria* healing practices include splashing holy water on the head for headaches, nerves, backaches, or tension. Incense is burned with herbs to cleanse the family and house. Herbal teas are believed to heal stomachaches but also to perform black magic and the evil use of powders is to put a hex on another.

In both *curanderismo* and *santeria*, sprays are used for a blessing or to remove a jinx. Seven African powders, dissolved in water, are used monthly to clean the house and rid it of spirits; one cleans from the front to the back door to drive spirits out the back. Holy water and candles also help; candles are lit to ask the saints for help. To secure aid from Santa Clara, one cleans oneself with egg and lights a white candle.

Today, religion continues to offer comfort and strength to H-L elders whose religious beliefs may differ from those of their younger relatives. Pain and suffering, a part of life, are often valued; they are seen as redemptive and as adding meaning to life. In old age, many elders return to earlier practices of their childhood faith (such as saying the rosary). If they have changed religions, they may unconsciously revert to Roman Catholic practices (such as using religious objects—icons, saints' pictures, an altar, candles). They may wish to burn candles in a hospital or a nursing home or put a scapula over a part of the body that is in pain (Rubio, 1995).

Psychosocial Tasks

There is little research on Erikson's psychosocial model (1950) with regard to H-Ls, but work on the development of minority-group children and consultations with H-L experts in the field have provided the following ideas. They will shed light on some of your elder H-L clients and on their relationships with children and grandchildren.

Hope (Trust versus Mistrust)

Yaniz (personal communication, 1995) said small H-L children are meant to be enjoyed, and babies are *engreidos* (more than elevated). Parents, wanting the best for a child, are overly responsive to the child's whims and desires; but that is because of a previously high rate of infant mortality. The parents want to be "good parents" so that the child "can stay." The *angelito* or *angelita* ("little angel") is God's gift, celebrated through baptism. Silva (personal communication, 1995) agreed that the quality of life is high at this stage—good foundation. Everyone is physically expressive with an infant.

Will (Autonomy versus Shame)

Often the seeds of interdependence are planted here. In the H-L family, this is not a matter of passive dependency or an unhealthy symbiosis but rather autonomy within the family. The H-L toddler's experience is different from that of the Anglo child—differences can be seen rhythmic patterns, role assignments, and parental expectations (Lar, 1973). While parents want children to be family-dependent, preschool Mexican-American children, for example, are expected to achieve *urbanidad*—success in human understanding and relationships and not necessarily in academics or finance (Wahab, 1973).

Yaniz (personal communication, 1995) said that exercising discipline is hard for some H-L parents who lack the necessary skills. Mother nurtures and rescues; Father is very strict; and so the parents are split. Mother says, "Wait until I tell your father; he will punish you," so Father appears uncaring and distant, though dedicated.

Purpose (Initiative versus Guilt)

Here, rigid gender differences emerge in choices of toys, games, and playmates. When school age approaches, the H-L child may encounter the first cultural conflicts as expectations of home and school vary—often resulting in an abrasive psychocultural adjustment. In 1983 Mejia wrote that Mexican-American children appeared to have more problems adapting to school, such as underachievement, cultural exclusion, marginality, discrimination, and impersonality.

Competence (Industry versus Inferiority)

Here, the child learns to be a worker. Yaniz said that about 5 percent of H-Ls make up the social upper class that tries to imitate royalty. The middle class is made up of professionals with work values similar to those of the United States. But in the lower class, the emphasis is on learning survival skills, learning to be tougher, clever, street-wise. H-L children learn to be industrious, Silva told me, but in a cooperative sense, around the home—not in a competitive sense in school or at work that might help them to fit into the United States.

Fidelity (Identity versus Diffusion)

Much of the work of self-identity takes place in adolescence. If teens such as Marita and Pepe Rodriguez reject their ethnicity—even their body type—their struggles for identity are difficult. Marita tried to find identity through . sex, Pepe through gang activities. For Carlos Hernandos, a dark Mexican, the message was that growing up Indian-looking and dark was not as good as growing up light and European-looking (Montalvo, 1991).

Yaniz said the Chicano movement started in the United States out of a painful sense of injustice and discrimination. Teens and young adults saw their parents deported, their property and language taken away, and they felt their elders had "sold out." But the civil rights movement helped them to discover who they were. It was a way to preserve identity and pride, as the barrios had been to their elders much earlier. Latino gangs, like Pepe's, offered a sense of belonging to a family that had its own rules, loyalties, and punishments.

Lopez (personal communication, 1995) said Chicano youths are angry that their elders are so powerless, and that serious culture and generation gaps exist. For example, young people hate having to be translators for older generations. Power, gained through drugs, and gangs offsets frustrations but breaks their elders' hearts.

Love (Intimacy versus Isolation)

Intimacy was never a goal in the H-L culture, Yaniz told me. "Spouses are private about hugging and kissing. You married to establish family roles, not to meet emotional needs from a spouse. Instead you had very close *compadres* who were extended family." Marital loyalty and fidelity are needed, but there is a double standard of sexual fidelity, he said: "Sexually unfaithful husbands may be accepted because they're loyal to family but an unfaithful woman is the worst kind."

Lopez said H-Ls didn't expect intimacy or closeness from marriage. Weddings are important, but they create separate lifestyles—though with much role security. A man's social life, the family and the *compadre* system, continues after marriage. A woman socializes with her children or sisters and tends not to have many friends or go out much. The more acculturated upper classes, however, handle intimacy much as Anglos do.

Yaniz said that H-L families are more united than separated. They tend to avoid confrontations, to gloss over problems, to hold the family together at all costs, and to present a united front to the world: "You can gossip about kin inside the family but not outside and you do not tolerate it from an outsider."

Care (Generativity versus Stagnation)

The older adult H-L doesn't "contribute to the community" in the sense that this phrase has in the United States. There are few H-L charities except for the church—which in Mexico is state-supported and survives without financial or volunteer help from members. Yaniz said that H-Ls give to charity, for example, in different ways: they may give a child to the priesthood or convent, and eventually these children will run institutions such as hospitals, orphanages, and Catholic youth groups.

Lopez said that H-Ls, being in general very hard workers, are sometimes simply too tired (or afraid) to contribute to their communities; volunteerism is a luxury. She said H-L elders volunteer all the time—in the family.

Hispanics value the group, stressing mutual empathy, sacrifice, conformity to expectations, and trust in members of the family and the community. True, this can demand individual sacrifices, but it promises prestige and respect. The trait known as *simpatia* indicates this strong group orientation: Respect and agreeableness are given and reciprocated; confrontation is avoided and discouraged.

Wisdom (Integrity versus Despair)

For many H-Ls, an important part of being parent is the prospect of becoming a grandparent. Grandparents often raise their own and others' grandchildren. This sense of hospitality in a large family—"the door is always open"—is not even a moral obligation; it is just something one does, Yaniz said. H-L children seek refuge with grandparents, but a problem arises when another culture is introduced. The child's language and behaviors may differ, creating culture shock.

When I asked H-L providers about "life satisfaction" among elders, Neville (personal communication, 1995) said she saw much dependency and dissatisfaction, and a feeling among elders that their children were not doing enough for them. She lamented that it is hard to form a network or neighborhood watch at a housing project. Reginato (personal communication, 1955) also noted much dependency among first-generation H-Ls, though less among the more acculturated. But what worried him most was a specific kind of depression he saw: Elders were not suicidal in earnest but did often say that they wished they were dead. He noted, "They seem to have given up and were only passive observers of life." Lopez (personal communication, 1995) said H-L older people wanted to participate in more activities but had to care for grandchildren and would not leave them with strangers. Also, they would like to live in senior housing, but their families needed their Social Security checks. All this led to isolation from their peers and to social withdrawal.

Many cultural influences add to the strengths of H-L elders. Hispanic "fatalism" is neither positive nor negative but more an acceptance of human frailties. Wisdom is recognizing limitations and having the courage to cope with them. In aging especially, H-L religious beliefs and customs support the concept of struggle as a normal part of being human.

The Subset Systems

The Ethnic Lens, layered onto the Gero Chi Model, implies substantial changes in the biopsychosocial systems of our H-L geroclients and their families.

The Biological System

In 1992, the life expectancy among H-Ls was 69.6 for men and 77.1 for women—lower than that of whites but higher than that of blacks. Heart disease, diabetes, and cancer were the principal killers. One in three elders (28.7 percent) had high blood pressure (the problem being greatest for Mexican men). H-Ls are estimated to be 300 percent more prone to non-insulin-dependent diabetes than the general population; and they have a higher-than-average incidence of most cancers (Villa, Cuellar, Gamel, & Yeo, 1993).

There is also a higher prevalence of arthritis among older Mexican Americans. H-L women are more likely to suffer from multiple illnesses such as hardening of the arteries, high blood pressure, cancer, and arthritis; men have more strokes. Several of these diseases are related to a lifestyle that includes obesity, malnutrition, little exercise, and high alcohol consumption among males (Villa et al., 1993).

In 1986, 41.2 percent of H-L elders reported poor to fair health, with high rates of disability. Of minorities, more have ADL problems; black and H-L elders need the greatest amount of household help. Fewer H-Ls had health insurance coverage, and H-Ls averaged fewer visits to doctors and less use of public health services than blacks or whites.

Along with low income and language problems, cultural factors are evidently a cause of underutilization of medical care. Self-diagnosis and self-treatment are prevalent because of a distrust of modern medicine among more traditional elders. In Mexico, the physician is esteemed—like a priest—but here in the United States the physician's advice may be merged with old-country beliefs and over-the-counter medications (OTCs), because the doctor and established medications are costly (Lopez, personal communication, 1995). Many H-L women believe that the sexual life is over by age 35 and that only a husband should view a woman's body; sexuality is a taboo subject, even medically. Thus few have breast or pelvic exams, according to Lopez. Underutilization is also linked to a close-knit family that likes to provide its own support. However, other observers argue that cultural explanations obscure the real issue: that H-L elders have a difficult time accessing the formal health system and therefore must rely on informal help instead.

H-L folk medicine is a synthesis of Spanish and Aztec ideas. The

Aztecs envisioned a balance of universal opposites: night-day, good-bad, hot-cold. In early times, Spaniards adhered to Greek and Roman theories: they saw the body as consisting of blood, phlegm, black bile, and yellow bile, each with hot-cold, wet-dry qualities. The unhealthy body was out of balance, but balance could be restored with treatments such as bloodletting, cupping, herbs, and poultices. Blood, passed on through families, determined one's destiny and explained one's powerlessness.

Ideas about old H-L diseases such as *empacho, mal ojo, susto, ateques de nervios, embrujaco,* and *bilis* vary in their importance today, but since they are said to affect soul, body, and mind, they—like beliefs about health—are a bridge·to the H-L psychological system.

Empacho develops when saliva is stuck in the stomach, causing vomiting, constipation, bloating, diarrhea, anorexia, and chills or fever. It is said to be related to poor diet, malnutrition, or stress incurred when eating with the family. A *santiguador* cures it with tea, diet, or a laxative prayer, or by massaging the stomach with an egg to loosen the blockage.

It is estimated that over half of H-L families have used folk remedies for *empacho* after seeing a physician. Some cures, considered harmful especially for children, can cause lead poisoning and other poisoning (Marsh & Hentges, 1988).

The symptoms of *Mal ojo* (evil eye) are headaches, insomnia, drowsiness, restlessness, fever, and vomiting and thought to be fatal. *Mal ojo* is said to be caused by disturbing relationships; children and women are most susceptible. The cure involves rubbing the body with an egg or touching the patient's head.

Susto (fright) occurs with loss of soul, and the cure is to coax the soul back through prayer, body massage, spitting cold water onto the patient, or sweeping the body. Family and cognitive counseling are also used.

Ataques de nervios (nervous attacks) occur after natural disasters and causes uncontrollable shouting, trembling, heart palpitations, heat from chest to head, fainting, and seizures—often at funerals or accidents, or during family arguments or fights. Recovery is rapid and the patient does not remember the *ataque.*

Ataques were seen in the 1950s among Puerto Ricans in the military. This malady later came to be known as a culturally derived syndrome, "an expression of anger and grief resulting from the disrupting of family systems, the process of migration, and concerns about family members in [the] country of origin" (Guarnaccia, De La Cancela, & Carrillo, 1989, p. 47).

Embrujado is a set of folk-defined conditions and interventions. Symptoms include hallucinations, anxiety, paranoid reactions, possession by spirits, witchcraft, and communication with supernatural beings. The overwhelmed victim is powerless to manage affairs and act appropriately. Bodily pains and deviant sexual behaviors are blamed on witches.

Bilis results from fantasies of revenge after a person has been badly treated by another or has been oppressed. Bile boils into the bloodstream, causing anxiety, vomiting, diarrhea, dizziness, migraine headaches, nightmares, loss of appetite, and urinary problems. The imbalance of yellow bile is caused by strong feelings: *susto* (anxiety), *tristeza* (sadness), and *envidia* (envy). *Bilis* is male-related; *susto* is female-related.

The Psychological System

Life satisfaction is reported to be good by most elders in the United States, but not, in general, by older H-Ls. Over half, mostly those with poor health and low income—and particularly those who immigrated in late adulthood—have reported little life satisfaction and spoke of extreme, serious problems (Andrews, Lyons, & Rowland, 1992). Angel and Angel (1992) reported that Cubans in ethnic ghettoes had higher life satisfaction than Mexicans or Puerto Ricans.

Depression

Research findings on depression among H-Ls are mixed. Rates are very high—especially for women and for people who are divorced, separated, age 75 and over, and with secondary or higher education (Morton, Schoenrock, Stanford, Peddecord, & Molgaard, 1990). However, Markides and Martin (1990) saw little correlation between divorce and depression, challenging the idea that the H-L family is an automatic protection from emotional problems. Positive marital interaction declined in old age, they said, because women do not consider divorce an option and find few substitutes for the discontinued role of mother.

Among H-L elders, affective disorders were strongly correlated with medical disabilities and dementia; Kemp, Staples, and Lopez-Aqueres (1987) linked these disorders to being female, poor, widowed, lonely, a caregiver, and monolingual (in Spanish). The lack of documented treatment of H-L elders with depression suggests that it goes unrecognized, perhaps because of a tendency to somatize psychological problems.

More acculturated United States-born elders appear to have less depression; abandoning some Mexican culture and incorporating aspects of the dominant society did not result in increased stress and did lower rates of depression (Zamanian, Thackery, Starrett, Brown, Lossman, & Blanchard,, 1992).

Dementia

There are few data on dementia among H-Ls. Physical markers confirming the disease and trained Spanish-speaking researchers are sparse. Many H-Ls do not recognize Alzheimer's disease, seeing it rather as a normal failing with aging and a return to childhood. The Spanish-Speaking Alzheimer's Disease Research Program (SSADRP) was created in 1986 to ensure inclusion of elderly Hispanics in epidemiological studies.

Valverde (personal communication, 1995) found that many rural clients around Salinas, California, viewed dementias as *mal ojo*— the evil eye or a curse, a cross to carry as punishment for one's sins or to obtain admission to heaven, as Alicia Perez saw it. Others prefer to think it is temporary, resulting from a problem with nerves or from not eating right. Some believe that the patient is revengeful or that the brain is drying up. Some families blame themselves for the impairment and spend much money on medications sold at the Mexican border, where they are cheaper or more available, to treat the disease. Still others seek *curanderos*.

Professionals agree that it is hard enough to diagnose Alzheimer's disease in the general population, but the task is enormous when one adds another language, high costs, a lack of convenient transportation for medical evaluations, and a dearth of culturally sensitive research tools to problems of an uninformed, often superstitious, and often shame-laden population (as in the case of Maria Martinez and Lily Rivas) who are reluctant to discuss private family matters. Taussig (1994) wrote,

I judge that Hispanic caregivers suffer from the same basic problems as their Anglo counterparts. I can tell you that this population may be suffering even more because of its lack of knowledge of the disease, its economic conditions, and the many different family compositions and situations related to emigration. (1994, p 69).

Alcoholism

Hispanics have higher rates of alcohol-related problems than the general population, but little is known about the alcoholic H-L (Lopez-Bushnell, Tyra, & Futrell, 1992). Many, like Antonio Gonzalez, do not see alcoholism as a medical problem. Rates do decrease with age, though. Older H-L women, who have little access to the mental health system, have very low rates, but some may hide their use of alcohol to relieve anxiety. Alcohol use by women rises with acculturation and education (Markides, Raky, Strou-Benham, & Trevino, 1990).

Barriers to Mental Health Services

Barriers are (1) financial, due to low income, lack of health insurance, ineligibility for Medicaid, and inability to pay for Medicare Part B; and (2) institutional—understaffed facilities, racial discrimination, high fees, cultural insensitivity, communication problems, inaccessible location, and lack of transportation. A barrier is also created when someone like Lily Rivas sees problems as a "cross to bear."

Strengths

Most H-L elders, even if they are poorly educated, have much common sense, sometimes stemming from an agrarian background, and are still respected by the young. Some ways of coping commonly seen among elders are religion; home remedies; reliance on family, friends, and compadres; folkways; selective ignoring; and learned helplessness. Felicia Marquez dogmatically insisted on getting help from her family—or none at all. Some people resort to passive-aggressive behavior, withdrawal when angry, and using folk wisdom to rationalize suffering as salvation. None of these methods are necessarily maladaptive unless overused. Despite the stereotype of dependency and passivity, Hispanic elders "rely on themselves to solve their mental health problems more often than they use the church, physician, or professional" (Starret, Rogers, & Decker, 1992).

The Sociological System

In H-L cultures, the family group supersedes the individual and the individual supports the group. *Personalismo,* a culturally recognized social style, stresses warm relationships, a strong personal commitment to others, and social status based on one's behavior with family or one's position in a formal institution. It is a paternalistic hierarchy, with *machismo* dictating male authority and female compliance. Divisions of labor and power by age and gender are well-defined and meaningful. Intelligence, education, and wealth are valued; teachers, healers, priests, males, and the aged rank highly. But this is also a young, reproducing society that soon will be a demographic majority in many areas in the United States. The emerging H-L population has less education and job skills than whites, and when the baby boomers reach old age (around 2010–2020), the bulk of the low-paid H-Ls and others will be supporting them. Some fear that racial and generational problems of a new magnitude will develop (Torres-Gil, 1986.)

The family is almost sacred, but there are indicators of some breakdown as H-Ls embrace a United States culture that does not expect the family to care for its elders. Family reciprocity is weakening as some young Chicanos, passing as whites, move on, leaving elders isolated and financially insecure. Elders, even those not at risk, fear to seek outside help, for various reasons. They may be reacting to recent anti-immigrant sentiment affecting citizenship and services, and they may also be reluctant to burden the young. Many have stopped answering their doorbells. Ironically, if the family meets all of an elder's needs, he or she may become lonely and isolated from peers, and thus even more dependent on the family.

But family support of elders is still a value in H-L cultures, and a highly interactive support network continues to exist (Markides & Martin, 1990.) Many elders reciprocate by sharing their homes and Social Security benefits, and by baby-sitting. Over 36 percent care for family children, and most will not pursue social services unless child care is provided (Andrews, 1989).

In Sotomayor's study of a barrio in Denver, most Chicano elders (80 percent) had much authority and responsibility for rearing grandchildren, teaching the culture, and keeping the family together with emotional support, advice, meals, and often money. In return, they received more esteem—especially the females, unless the grandfather was still employed. Retirement because of poor health was less traumatic for females, who continued contributing at home (Maldanado, 1985).

Friends continue to be important in old age. The *compadre* system of best friends among males extends the family. *Compradazgo* is the extended honorary family structure of godparents who ensure the welfare and religious education of children—sometimes with financial support.

Caregiving can mean support with congeniality or support with conflict. The H-L caregiver is often an unassisted, depressed female, not empowered with much information. As in the Mexican movie *Como Agua Para Chocolate*, the caregiving role is determined by sex and by one's place in the family. Sometimes the caregiver is the oldest daughter, the unmarried daughter, or the youngest daughter; a violation of the general rule is considered bad. Adult children were the main source of support for H-L elders, female children helping with personal problems and health matters and males with finances and home repairs and upkeep (Markides & Martin, 1990).

In a study in Tampa, Florida, Cuban, Spanish, and Puerto Rican caregivers were assigned to their roles by gender. Daughters, daughters-in-law, and female nonrelatives handled the primary burden and, like Lily Rivas, they often bore the stigma of the demented elder's "craziness" (Henderson & Gutierrez-Mayka, 1992). Older caregivers were less likely than younger ones to accept support sessions. In another study, out of 17 Mexican American caregivers for Alzheimer's patients in San Jose, only one was sharing the burden (Villa et al., 1993).

Reluctance to seek help often results in depression. Gallagher-Thompson (personal communication, 1995) said that a daughter is often pushed into a stressful solo caregiving role with no help from her siblings, even if they are nearby. Asking for help is considered aggressive; instead, the caregiver becomes depressed. Puerto Rican caregivers also showed a high rate of depressive symptoms; the majority could get no respite or help from their network for what they saw as their filial obligation (Cox & Monk, 1993).

Valverde (personal communication, 1995) believes that male spouses are often loyal caregivers because of the *machismo* value of protectiveness. A man will usually refuse placement for his wife, feeling a commitment to protect her. Wives, accustomed to a motherly role that nurtures and then lets go, find placement of a spouse easier, Valverde said. Yaniz (personal communication, 1995) thinks that H-L males, lacking nurturing skills, made poor caregivers. Lopez (1995) concurs: "If mother has a crisis, he'll call the children . . . but at least he'll call."

When loved ones die, Catholic H-Ls usually pray for their souls in monthly, then yearly novenas. On All Souls' Day, special observances are held with prayers, cemetery visitations, and grave decorations.

Owing to a long history of tragedies, dying causes little fear, Yaniz says. Saying good-bye is usually done with mariarchis, marigolds, and an optimistic belief in an afterlife, *las golondrinas,* which says, "You are the swallow that can go to different skies and one day will return."

Aging Tasks

Tasks of aging are the same for the H-L as for the general population, but they are perhaps more difficult to achieve because of the issues described in the Ethnic Lens. In some cases, the task of independence and assertive control must be altered to include the value of interdependence; and control may be more a family matter than an individual matter.

As with AI/ANs, we must add another task, the maintenance of continued harmony of the ethnic culture and the dominant cultures, so that one's final days can be spent in comfort and dignity without despair. But whether and how much anyone chooses to acculturate or assimilate is a personal choice.

EXERCISE

Think again of the H-L examples. After applying the H-L Gero Chi Lens, what new knowledge about H-Ls contributes to your understanding of these elders and their families? What more do you need to know?

Chapter 9

H-Ls and Gerocounseling

Now we will layer the H-L Ethnic Lens onto the Gerocounseling Model in order to provide culturally sensitive services to H-L elders and their families. The Ethnic Lens and the Gero Chi Lens should help us to assess and incorporate the H-L family's traditions in regard to ethics, relationships, communication, and seeking help. You will find that the gerocounseling of H-L elders and their families takes on special nuances and requires some unique approaches.

Generic Ethnogerocounseling

Ethics Skills

Ethics in gerocounseling entails a commitment to three principles: autonomy, beneficence, and fidelity. Each should be maintained unless there is a stronger, overriding moral obligation to do otherwise. In ethnogerocounseling, this occurs often, as in the following examples.

> On his way to work, Maurio Sanchez dropped off his mother and sister, Rose, at the hospital. Since Mrs. Sanchez was to have minor surgery that day, it was necessary for her to sign informed consent

forms, but neither she nor Rose spoke English. Also, Maurio made all the big family decisions.

Mr. Gonzales is near death, and his entire extended family wishes to rally around him to pray for his soul. Grandchildren want to give him a final kiss. The facility's rule is "no children" and "only two visitors at a time." The family also wants to light vigil candles, but the rule is "no fires."

June L., a social worker, was called in because Maria M. was noncompliant and refused baths. June didn't understand Spanish but figured out that Maria needed a scapular to "make the sickness go away." June decided that Maria was not only noncompliant but delusional and required psychiatry.

Carmen P., new to the United States and homesick, baby-sat daily with her grandchildren. Learning about a senior lunch program, she took the children and shared her lunch with them. She was told that federal regulations forbade feeding children in a seniors-only program. Carmen stopped going.

Cultural sensitivity can prevent such "iatrogenic" problems or expedite solutions. Mrs. Sanchez's doctor's aide could have arranged a time for Maurio to sign readied forms in advance, since he could not afford to take time off from work. Maurio could have been advised to tell his mother that it was okay to put her "X" on the form. Or, if Mrs. Sanchez needed special help, a reliable interpreter could have been used.

Knowing H-L customs about death and dying, the staff could place Mr. Gonzalez in an end room across from a lounge where the family could "camp out." The rules about children and number of visitors could be bent if the good of the patient, not the convenience of the facility, is the primary consideration. If lighted candles are not allowed, the family might be advised to purchase electric candles, or the facility could have wired candles on hand.

With cultural awareness, June L. could have taught the staff about a Catholic scapular, how to protect it in a small plastic bag, and how to put it to one side when bathing a patient.

The senior center should know that taking care of grandchildren is a priority for H-Ls. Perhaps a special fund drive could be undertaken to raise money for children's food.

Consuela N. is being psychologically abused by her partner. He controls her, cavorts with campadres, uses needed family money for liquor, and does not let her visit her sisters. Counsuela is depressed but will not leave him.

Granting autonomy means not imposing your own values. You may be critical of the traditional H-L system regarding gender roles, but don't impose your egalitarianism on H-L women under the guise of beneficence. That may create even greater stress, because change can be harmful if it is not affirmed by the culture. But feminist Latina counseling with a sociocultural perspective that offers support groups, reframing gender and mothering roles, and opportunities to learn how traumatic events can lead to somatization have been successful (Comas-Diaz, 1987).

Relationship Skills

Along with culturally sensitive ethics, your relationship skills need to take on some new slants with H-Ls.

Ease into Rapport

At first, H-Ls are usually formal, polite, and reserved, and you will follow this lead by addressing them formally, using last names for yourself and all adults present. Your geroclient will pay some attention to your education but more to your "calling" (Maduro, 1983). But once rapport is established, there may be hugging, touching, and impromptu visits, as "friendship" becomes "kinship."

Use an Open Approach

Shake hands warmly. The H-L expects active, two-way participation characterized by *personalismo*—the inclination to relate to and trust individuals instead of formal organizations. Therefore, in working with H-Ls—unlike working with others—the gerocounselor functions both as a person and as an agency representative.

Take Your Time

Again, develop *personalismo*. Show a social interest in the geroclient before becoming involved in procedures. To prevent distrust and defensiveness, avoid direct questions and don't expect full disclosure. Be warm, use humor, and praise accomplishments and clever statements while keeping an appropriate distance. And, of course, be playful with the children.

Be Creative

Falicov (1982) suggested using culture-specific structural and strategic counseling. Your powerful role can be diffused by your becoming a "philosopher of life," telling stories and anecdotes. Use humor, analogies, proverbs, popular songs, or what Falicov called "a mysterious, unexpected communication that transmits an existential sense of the absurd, the impossibility to win, or the reversals that life plays in consonance with Mexican cultural themes (p. 149).

"Treating Cubans," Hernandez (1992) wrote, "as one would treat other Hispanic groups or even other minority groups is not going to work because Cubans do not consider themselves 'Victims of Society' nor do elderly Cubans consider themselves a minority group" (p. 56). They retain their sense of peoplehood even though later Cuban immigrants gave up many cultural modes and beliefs about the extended family and Catholicism.

Use Countertransference

Countertransference is used positively by giving feedback about what the counselor is thinking, feeling, and even fantasizing; but do not use self-disclosure or trivia inappropriately. Maduro (1983) suggests that counselors not make an issue of their ignorance when asking about cultural norms for this could increase their authority or create a cultural distance. A safe question would be, "What do you believe elderly people should do when they can no longer take care of themselves safely?"

Use Transference

Your elder clients may come with distrust as a result of years of discrimination; but in the pecking order of the downtrodden, they too may have prejudices about other groups. Thus your own ethnic or racial background may be a target. When issues of transference surface, a frank discussion is necessary. Try not to take it personally, be nonjudgmental, and offer another counselor if that seems indicated. When no other counselor is possible, it may be effective to treat the client like any other difficult client, who may be won over with "TLC" and positive perseverance.

Communication Skills

An emotive, dramatic tone is better than an efficient, highly structured approach. When possible, use the language your client communicates in most comfortably, realizing that people who are emotionally upset or undergoing a crisis do not communicate well in a second or third language. People are most able to express emotions in their native tongue—particularly if it is Spanish, a colorful, emotive language where there is little distinction between formality and informality. A client's stumbling English may lead to misdiagnosed anxiety or inexpressiveness.

Rodreiguz (personal communication, 1995) stressed using culturally sensitive materials in Spanish. She showed me some *Foto Novelas*, soap opera–like comic books about families coping with Alzheimer's disease. Many multilingual educational materials can be obtained from the Alzheimer's Association, the National Institute on Aging, and AARP, as well as from H-L organizations.

Learn how to use interpreters. It is often not a good idea to use relatives especially children. But when relatives are making the decisions about health care, it is imperative to include them.

Active Questioning

Don't assume. When you are trying to elicit feelings, ask the H-L to explain. If feelings are expressed in bodily terms (such as "the heart hurts") know the feeling usually identified with each body part. Pressing for personal disclosure or a baring of the client's soul, or professing your own interpretations of nonverbal behaviors, may be too much.

Active Listening

Watch for too much agreement. "Mexicans have a hundred ways of saying no without ever saying it," Falicov wrote (1982, p. 153). If they are quiet, don't assume that they are agreeing; encourage feedback.

Check to determine whether differences in communication are cultural or dysfunctional. For example, you may encourage clients to use "I" sentences and to "own" their feelings or their behaviors. But H-Ls, as part of *personalismo,* are socialized to use *indirectas,* an indirect approach, as a matter of courtesy. The H-L elder is apt to say, "One doesn't do that" or "Some people feel that way."

Ethnogerocounseling Assessment

Assessment, facilitated by the H-L Ethnic Lens and the Gero Chi Lens, leads to an understanding of your H-L clients. After rapport is established, you will probably begin by discussing the presenting problems and then moving on to explore your client's immigration or migration patterns (Falicov, 1982). You might say, "I know you're here because of a difficulty with the people next door, but first tell me a little about yourself. How long have you lived here, and where did you come from originally?"

Caution! Tread lightly here. Such questions, in today's anti-immigrant climate, might make your client suspicious, defensive, or secretive; you might be seen as another bureaucrat inquiring about illegal status. Your geroclient may be "legal," but his or her relatives may not be—or suspiciousness may be just an instinctive reaction.

It is imperative to keep abreast of current immigration laws and regulations so that you may act responsibly and, it is hoped, in the client's best interests. Sometimes it is better not to know about a client's status. If you do know, ensure confidentiality when possible. As a first intervention, you may offer information about agency or governmental policies and where to get legal advice.

However, immigration patterns will tell you about a client's degree of acculturation, stressors, family splits and alliances, losses and gains, and strengths and resiliency; all this will help in the formulation of a care plan. Falicov (1982) advised not to get bogged down with details and dates initially but to be sympathetic about the plight of the immigrant family and even share your own experiences, if applicable, on a nonspecific level.

A genogram breaks the ice and supplies valuable information (Burlingame, 1995). Along with data about immigration, it reveals the nature of the informal support system and the closeness of the extended, nuclear, and fictive-kin family; and it helps you to decide, with the elder, who should attend family sessions. Questions about timing are important because they reveal the duration of the problem, the history of losses, and the client's memory and orientation.

Asking, "Why does this problem exist?" and "How did you deal with things like this in the past?" can lead to clues about cultural health-related beliefs and practices and provide procedural guidance.

Assessment instruments such as the Katz Index of Activities of Daily Living (ADL), the Minnesota Multiphasic Personality Inventory (MMPI), the Mini-Mental State Examination (MMSE), and the Geriatric Depression Scale (GSD) are now available in Spanish. But this does not necessarily mean that they have been culturally correlated to fit your client, who may be illiterate, newly arrived, or not acculturated. Attempts to validate Spanish versions are in the infant stage.

Look at the whole picture. In your assessment, consider neighborhood conditions, such as ethnic social opportunities, accessibility of transportation and services, crime rates, and gang activity. Fear and suspiciousness may be not paranoia but realistic responses to being hounded by creditors or immigration officers, or victimized by crime on the street. A complete physical exam may reveal that exposure to pesticides or agricultural chemicals is causing mental symptoms. Estrangement from loved ones may be creating situational, not clinical, depression.

Ethnogerocounseling Goals

While the solution of the presenting problem will be an immediate goal, empowerment of the H-L will be your ultimate goal. In setting goals, don't overlook culture.

One goal might be to incorporate *curanderismo* and religion into a treatment plan, if appropriate, by bringing in a *curandero* or a priest to help.

Remember that bargaining is important in H-L culture. In Mexico, for instance, this interpersonal process is enjoyed by both tourists and sellers alike. Use this cultural habit by turning a goal into a bargain. For example, Mrs. Diaz agreed to go to a Spanish center if her daughter would pay her more attention by driving her there.

Choosing Ethnogerocounseling Modalities

In most cases, family counseling is the modality of choice for interdependent H-L elders. Before they came to you, your clients most likely tried ethnic remedies: support from family or *compadres*, advice from an older neighbor (a *señora* or *persona mayor*), or treatment from a folk healer. The elder (perhaps believing the problem is a punishment or unnatural victimization) and the family (trying to decide if it is natural or supernatural) may also be seeing a *curandera* or *curandero*. But, Maduro advised, you should know that family has been intimately involved all the way and that a cure always requires family participation (1983, p. 872).

It is helpful to see some family members separately for a few sessions. In sessions with the whole family, younger people, out of respect for their elders, may suppress certain facts and feelings. Or you may wish to put some space between an overbearing parent and a spousal relationship or to separate overly protective adult children whose devotion is preventing a parent from forming outside relationships. Explain to elders, who prize *familismo,* that these "breakouts" can strengthen siblings' solidarity and hence family solidarity.

Many H-Ls resist marital treatment unless they are at the brink of divorce. Even then, they may see a successful marriage as a matter of luck and a wise choice rather than something to be worked on. Also, with *indirectas,* spouses are not supposed to display anger. A woman may feel compelled to function more as a mother than as a sexual partner, and both partners may put the family over individual needs. But do not try to weaken the role of maternal self-sacrifice. Instead, use paradox; reframe that situation to show she is helping her children by strengthening her marriage. Since couples use children and *compadres* to compensate for a bad marriage, begin with a focus on family and friends (Falicov, 1982).

Families of lower socioeconomic status relate best to brief, problem-oriented approaches that redefine a situation in terms of current needs, cultural expectations, and practical realities. Structural family therapy emphasizing generational boundaries can be used (Haley, 1976; Minuchin, Montalvo, & Guerney, 1960).

Family counselors often try to bring to the surface some 'family secret' that may be contributing to a problem. Once it is out, the counselor wonders aloud why the secret is necessary to maintain the family balance. In H-L families, the secret may be a secondary gain from the problem, or it may be reinforcing the primary culture by bringing the family together. For example, grandmother may "need" to be ill to maintain family solidarity.

This may be especially true for Cuban families; Felicia Marquez, for instance, feels that her suffering may help her stay in control of her family's destiny and that her burden is her fate or her punishment. While this reasoning may smack of masochism to the white observer, it may contribute to Cubans' low suicide rates (Hernandez, 1992).

A total family approach may not work in Cuban families, because multiple generations are not as supportive. Hernandez (1992) recommended exploration of the Cuban family's migratory history, its degree of bilingualism, geographic locations of the extended family, strength of caregivers, degree of acculturation, and female roles. But, she added, Cubans are private people and may conceal family problems with excuses, a united front, projection, or denial of pain and problems. Desiring total secrecy, they do not want to discuss issues they consider shameful such as Alzheimer's disease (caused by bad blood), mental illness, AIDS, mental retardation, or sexually-transmitted diseases.

Pride is necessary; don't destroy it. Hernandez wrote that a Cuban woman will wear herself out cleaning before a service provider visits, feeling that she is a failure if her house is not spotless. But your job may be to help her observe doctor's orders to work less. Reframing the situation to relieve her anguish, you might say, "Senora, you have done your duty well as wife and mother, and now the doctor and your family want you to have the help you deserve. Household help will enable you to spend more time in prayer or being the grandmother that you want to be—which is right for now."

Interpretations of family dysfunction will cause insecurity and apathy; instead, search for strengths, give genuine praise, and give each family a sense of its own dignity (Falicov, 1982, p. 150).

Successful group counseling with H-Ls has been reported by

several authors. All stressed that recruitment and progress were facilitated by strict attention to cultural norms.

Ethnogerocounseling Interventions

Empowerment of H-L clients—the ultimate goal of counseling—has two parts: cognitive (providing information) and affective (offering emotional support). Ethnic elders need much information in order to function in the everyday affairs of this bewildering system, a task that is more difficult if there is a language handicap. One of your first interventions may be a referral for instruction in English, but some clients may not want to take on a second language, preferring to rely on the family.

Reframing has already been mentioned. This is a popular cognitive intervention that involves putting a situation in a different context so that the client may look at it in a fresh new way. It is especially useful in ethnogerocounseling when confrontation may not be advisable.

> Eva says that her husband Tony is bossy, but Eva is really the bossy one. Still, the culture supports males as the "boss." Alicia reframed this, saying, "Eva, I can see that while you are burdened with planning, Tony is still the boss of the house. He probably makes you do these things because you are best at them and he is so busy." Alicia's reframing did not take power and control away from Eva (which she desires to keep) but gives Eva an excuse for Tony and helps to maintain the cultural myth.

As noted earlier, Falicov (1982) wrote that while you would not tell an H-L that her wifely role was as important as her maternal role, you could reframe the counseling goal as "helping the children by strengthening the marriage."

The success of most interventions depends on support and encouragement which you give naturally. Sometimes, in a very difficult crisis, this can be a temporary crutch until former coping mechanisms reappear or new coping mechanisms develop. In aging, old coping strategies sometimes no longer work; and for ethnic elders in a new country, some old mechanisms are bound to become obsolete. Supportively, you will be mustering up old defenses and coping methods and also teaching new ones. Here, "life review" or "reminiscence" counseling can be helpful. The desirability of encouraging H-L elders to recall their home country and their experiences of immigration and migration has been stressed. Such travelogues validate a person's life and remind him or her of personal strengths and resiliency. They not only help an elder to make life experiences whole and to reach a sense of Eriksonian integrity; in most cases, they also reinforce the original culture as a strong support system.

Ethnogerocounseling Terminations

The end of the first session may be too soon to provide tentative impressions and goals, because many H-Ls are person-centered, not task-centered. Instead, praise the family for their ability to describe their problem and for caring enough to do something about it by coming. Keep any first goals or homework tasks simple—like bringing in more information about medications (a bagful or a list).

As you help this polite family, you will be appreciated and even acknowledged as kin. At termination, you may be invited for a meal or given a homemade gift. Do not suspect that transference has gone awry but see these gestures as part of the H-L elder's hospitable tradition.

Earlier sections discussed some H-L beliefs and practices regarding death and dying. When possible, any help that you as a provider can give to allow for a "good death" in a cultural sense is important. Rubio (1995) suggested that when possible, the dying patient wants to hear about the family and the world to maintain a connection. Proper respect and attention should be given to religious symbols and customs. Be tender with the patient, Rubio said, stroking and sympathetically listening to complaints about symptoms or the hospital staff. While truth is important in family planning, if a discussion of death is taboo and is believed to bring on the death itself, ask the eldest son for guidance.

If a priest is requested, call while the patient is still conscious and lucid. The dying person will want to make his or her confession and make peace with God and relatives. Often the family will say the rosary together. If the dying person has left the church, reassure him or her it is okay to say Catholic prayers.

After a death, the traditional H-L family will want time with the body. Ask for instructions about preparing the body, as customs vary. Often a female cleanses the body; a scapular is put around the neck and a rosary in the hands. Ask the family for instructions on closing the eyes; sometimes the eyelids are covered with a scarf, tape, or coins. Usually, candles are lit and a priest is present (Rubio, 1995).

Everyone is supposed to say good-bye, often with marigolds—the flower of mourning—and replicas of swallows returning to their true nests. Bereaved females, wearing black, and males, wearing black armbands, may hold on to their grief for two years—or forever. But many elder men feel compelled to remarry immediately, to replace the supporting spouse on whom they depended. AARP (1990) gave the following advice on grief:

> It is important to accept each person as [he or she is]. Determine how you can best help each individual. You may find that what one person needs most is person-to-person contact; another may need you most as a telephone contact, someone to call just to talk to during the night if [he or she] can't sleep. It could be that you provide a person with transportation to and from a support group. Whatever your role, if you move gently, it will serve a need and be appreciated. (pp. 15, 16)

EXERCISE

Think again of the elders who were described at the beginning of the H-L section. On the basis of some of the principles of ethnogerocounseling discussed here, how would you devise a care or treatment plan? How would you proceed? What more do you need to know? Include both micro and macro interventions.

References for Part III

Administration on Aging (1992). Educating hard-to-reach minority groups about Alzheimer's disease. *Aging Magazine*. Washington, DC: Administration on Aging.

Allende, I. (1993). *The Infinite Plan*. New York: HarperCollins.

American Association of Retired Persons (1990). *African•Asian•Hispanic•Native Indian Customs of Bereavement*. Washington, DC: AARP.

American Association of Retired Persons (1990). *Hispanic elders discuss health interests and needs*. Washington, DC: AARP.

American Association of Retired Persons Minority Affairs (1995). *A Portrait of older minorities*. Washington, DC: AARP.

American Society on Aging (1992). *Serving elders of color: Challenges to providers and the aging network*. San Francisco: American Society on Aging.

Andrews, J. (1989, September). Poverty and poor health among elderly Hispanic Americans. Baltimore, MD: Commonwealth Fund Commission on Elderly People Living Alone.

Andrews, J., Lyons, B., & Rowland, D. (1992). Life satisfaction and peace of mind: A comparative analysis of elderly Hispanic and other elderly Americans. *Clinical Gerontologist, 11,* 21–42.

Angel, J. & Angel, R. (1992). Age at migration, social connections, and well-being among elderly Hispanics. *Journal of Aging and Health, 4,* 480–499.

Bastida, E. & Juarez, R. (1991). Older Hispanic women: A decade in review. In M. Sotomayor (Ed.), *Empowering Hispanic families: A critical issue for the '90s*. Milwaukee, WI: Family Service of America, pp. 155–171.

Bernal, G. (1982). Cuban families. In M. McGoldrick, J. Pearce, & J. Giordano, *Ethnicity and family therapy*. New York: Guilford, pp. 187–207.

Buriel, R. (1984). Integration with traditional Mexican-American culture and sociocultural adjustment. In J. Martinez & R. Mendoza (Eds.), *Chicano psychology* (2nd ed.). New York: Academic.

Burlingame, V. (1995). *Gerocounseling: Counseling elders and their families*. New York: Springer.

Castez, G. (1994). Providing services to Hispanic/Latino populations: Profiles in divsersity. *Social Work 39* (3), 288–296.

Comas-Diaz, L. (1987). Feminist therapy with mainland Puerto Rican women. *Psychology of Women Quarterly 11,* 461–474.

Comas-Diaz, L., & Griffith, E. (Eds.). (1987). *Clinical guidelines in cross-cultural mental health*. New York: John Wiley.

Cox, C. & Monk, A. (1993). Black and Hispanic caregivers of dementia victims: Their needs and implications for services. In C. Barresi & D. Stull (Eds.), *Ethnic elderly and long-term care*. New York: Springer, pp. 56–57.

Facundo, J. (1991). Sensitive mental health services for low-income

Puerto Rican families. In M. Sotomayor (Ed.), *Empowering Hispanic families,* pp. 121–139.

Falicov, J. (1982). Mexican families. In M. McGoldrick, J. Pearce, & J. Giordano (Eds.), *Ethnicity and family therapy.* New York: Guilford, pp. 134–163.

Fowles, D. (1991). *A profile of older Americans: 1991.* Washington, DC: AARP.

Franklin, G. & Kaufman, K. (1982). Group psychotherapy for elderly female Hispanic outpatients. *Hospital and Community Psychiatry, 33* (5), 385–387.

Gallagher-Thompson, D., Arguello, D., Johnson, C., Talamantes, M., Arguello, T., Meyer, M., Moorehead, R. & Polich, T. (1991). *The process of developing "Anger Management" classes for Hispanic family caregivers.* Paper presented at the meeting of the Gerontological Society of America, San Francisco, CA.

Gallegos, J. (1991). Culturally relevant services for Hispanic elderly. In M. Sotomayor (Ed.), *Empowering Hispanic families,* pp. 121–139.

Garcia-Preto, N. (1982). Puerto Rican Families. In M. McGoldrick, J. Pearce, & J. Giordano (Eds.), *Ethnicity and family therapy.* New York: Guilford, pp. 164–186.

Gonzalez, G. (1991). Hispanics in the past two decades, Latinos in the next two: Hindsight and foresight. In M. Sotomayor (Ed.), *Empowering Hispanic families,* pp. 1–19.

Green, J. (1995). *Cultural awareness in the human services: A multi-ethnic approach.* Boston: Allyn and Bacon.

Guarnaccia, P., De La Cancela, V., & Carrillo, E. (1989). The multiple meanings of *ataques de nervios* in the Latino community. *Medical Anthropology 11,* 47–62.

Haley, J. (1976). Approaches to family therapy. In J. Haley (Ed.), *Changing families-A family therapy reader.* New York: Grune and Stratton.

Henderson, J., & Gutierrez-Mayka, M. (1992). Ethnocultural themes: Caregiving to Alzheimer's disease patients in Hispanic families. In T. Brink (Ed.), *Hispanic Aged Mental Health.* New York: Hayworth.

Hernandez, G. (1992). *The family and its aged members: the Cuban experience.* New York: Hayworth.

Keefe, S., & Padilla, A. (1987). *Chicano Ethnicity.* Albuquerque: University of New Mexico Press.

Kemp, B., Staples, F., & Lopez-Aqueres, W. (1987). Epidemiology of depression and dysphoria in our elderly Hispanic population: Prevalence and correlates. *Journal of the American Geriatric Society, 35,* 920–926.

Kittler, P., & Sucher, K. (1989). *Food and culture in America*. New York: Van Nostrand and Reinhold.

Korte, A. (1978). *Social interaction and morals of Spanish-speaking elderly*. Unpublished dissertation. University of Denver, Colorado.

Koss-Chioino, J., & Canive, J. (1993). The interaction of popular and clinical diagnostic labeling: The case of *embrujado*. *Medical Anthropology 15*, 171–188.

Lar, R. (1973). *A cross-cultural study of infant movement and pre-verbalization behavior*. Unpublished dissertation, University of California at Irvine.

Lopez, C., & Aguilera, E. (1991). On the sidelines: Hispanic elderly and the continuum of care. Washington, DC: Policy Analysis Center and Office of Institutional Development.

Lopez-Bushnell, F., Tyra, P., & Futrell, M. (1992). Alcoholism and the Hispanic older adult. In T. Brink (Ed.), *Hispanic aged mental health*. New York: Hayworth.

Maduro, R. (1983). Curanderismo and Latino views of disease and curing. *Western Journal of Medicine, 139*, 868–874.

Maldonado, D. (1985). The Hispanic elderly: A socio-historical framework for public policy. *Journal of Applied Gerontology, 4* (1), 18–27.

Maldono-Dennis, M. (1969). *Puerto Rico: Una interpretacion historico social*. Mexico, DF: Siglo XXI Editores.

Markides, K., & Krause, N. (1985). Intergenerational solidarity and psychological well-being among older Mexican Americans: A three-generations study. *Journal of Gerontology, 40* 390–392.

Markides, K., & Martin, H. (1990). *Selected findings from two San Antonio, TX studies: Older Mexican Americans*. San Antonio: Tomas Rivera Center.

Markides, K., Raky, L., Stroup-Benham, C., & Trevino, F. (1990). Acculturation and alcohol consumption in the Mexican population of the southwestern United States: Findings from HHANES 1888. 84. *American Journal of Public Health, 80* (Suppl.), 42–46.

Marsh, W., & Hentges, K.(1988). Mexican folk remedies and conventional medical care. *American Family Physician, 37*, 257–262.

Mejia, D. (1983). The development of Mexican-American children. In G. Powell (Ed.), *The psychosocial development of minority children*. New York: Brunner/Mazel, pp. 77–114.

Minuchin, S., Montalvo, B., & Guerney, B. (1960). *Families of the slums: An exploration of their treatment*. New York: Basic.

Monahan, D., Greene, V., & Coleman, P. (1991). Caregiver support groups: Factors affecting use of services. *Gerontologist, 31,* Special Issue II, 100.

Montalvo, F. (1991). Phenotyping, acculturation, and biracial assimilation of Mexican-Americans. In M. Sotomayor (Ed.), *Empowering Hispanic families,* pp. 97–120.

Morton, D., Schoenrock, S., Stanford, E., Peddecord, K., & Molgaard, C. (1989). Use of the CES-D among a community sample of old Mexican Americans. *Journal of Cross-cultural Gerontology, 4,* 289–306.

Newton, F., & Ruiz, R. (1980). Chicano culture and mental health among the elderly. In M. Miranda & R. Ruiz (Eds.), *Chicano aging and mental health.* Rockville, MD: U.S. Dept. of Health and Human Services, NIMH, pp. 38–75.

Rubio, Jose (1995, March). Spiritual concerns of the dying. Presented at Cultural Diversity and End of Life Issues Conference at Stanford University: Palo Alto, CA: Stanford Geriatric Education Center.

Sotomayor, M. (Ed.) (1991). *Empowering Hispanic families: A critical issue for the '90s.* Milwaukee, Wi: Family Service of America.

Sotomayor, M., & Curiel, H. (1988). *Hispanic elderly: A cultural signature.* Edinburg, TX: Pan American University Press.

Starrett, R., Rogers, D., & Decker, J. (1992). The self-reliance behavior of the Hispanic elderly in comparison to their use of formal mental health helping networks. In T. Brink (Ed.), *Hispanic aged mental health.* New York: Hayworth, pp. 157–169.

Taussig, I. (1994, September 16). Alzheimer's disease and the Hispanic older adult. Paper presented at the Ethnicity and Dementias Conference, Stanford University, Palo Alto, CA.

Taussig, I., & Trejo, L. (1992). Outreach to Spanish-speaking caregivers of persons with memory impairments: A brief report. In T. Brink (Ed.), *Hispanic aged mental health.* New York: Hayworth, pp. 183–189.

Torres-Gil, F. (Ed.) (1986). *Hispanics in an aging society.* New York: Aging Society Project of Carnegie Corporation.

U.S. Bureau of the Census. (1990, May). *The Hispanic Population in the United States.* March 1989, Current Population Reports, Series P.020, No. 444. Washington, DC: U.S. Government Printing Office.

U.S. Department of Health and Human Services. (1990, April). *SSA/90 Annual Report to Congress.* Washington, DC: Social Security Administration.

Vega, W., Hough, R., & Romero, A. (1983). Family life patterns of

Mexican-Americans. In G. Powell (Ed.), *The psychosocial development of minority group children*. New York: Brunner/Mazel, pp. 194–215.

Villa, M., Cuellar, J., Gamel, N., & Yeo, G. (1993). *Aging and health: Hispanic American elders* (2nd ed.). Palo Alto, CA: Stanford Geriatric Education Center.

Wahab, Z. (1973, November 28–December 2). Barrio school: White school in a brown country. Paper presented at the Annual Convention of the American Anthropological Association, New Orleans, LA. ERIC, ED092294.

Zamanian, K., Thackery, M., Starrett, R., Brown, L., Lassman, D., & Blanchard, A. (1992). Acculturation and depression in Mexican American elderly. In T. Brink (Ed.), *Hispanic aged mental health*. New York: Hayworth, pp. 109–121.

Acknowledgments for Part III

I thank the Geriatric Education Centers at Stanford University in Palo Alto, Calif., and Marquette University in Milwaukee, Wisconsin, for generously sharing hard-to-get current literature on ethnicity, aging, and Hispanic-Latino American families. Many individuals also helped in the preparation of this chapter.

I wish to thank the H-L health and social service providers who took time out of their busy schedules to grant me interviews.

From California: Michele Bjerke, MA, and Daniel Reginato, MSW, from the Mexican American Community Services Agency, Inc.; Ruth Lopez from the San Benito Health Foundation; Veronica Rodriguez, MSW, from the Greater San Francisco Bay Area; Irene Valverde, Celine Ossinalde, and Maria Yanez from the Monterrey County Alzheimer's Association; Margarita Nevel from the Oakland Spanish Speaking Unity Council; Alicia Saucedo Marquez, PhD candidate in Daly City; Juliette S. Silva, PhD, from the College of Social Work at San Jose State University; Manuel Yaniz, PhD, at the Gardner Health Center, San Jose; and Dolores Gallagher-Thompson, PhD, VA Hospital, Menlo Park.

From New York City: Rebecca Carel, CSW, and Carmen Nunez, MA at the Fort Washington Houses Services for the Elderly and the Bilingual Access Specialists Miriam Roldan and Karen Argueta at the Instituto Puertorriqueno/Hispano Para Peronas Mayores. From Florida: Margarita Longaria, SW, and Sylvia Thompson, SW, Supervisor, at the Palm Beach County Division of Senior Services, and Lyanne Azqueta, MA, at Hanley-Hazelden, West Palm Beach.

And from Wisconsin: Carmen M. Rigau, MS, ESL, and Adult Education Counselor, Gateway Technical School, Racine: Juan Torres, Kenosha County Alcohol and Drug Council, and Vanda Kinderman, United Migrant Opportunity Services (UMOS), in Kenosha; Ramon Olveda, Retired and Volunteer. From Texas: Dolores Espadas Wilson, Retired and Volunteer.

PART IV

African American (AA) Elders

> After the Egyptian and Indian, the Greek and Roman, the Teuton and Mongolian, the Negro is a sort of seventh son, born with a veil, and gifted with second-sight in this American world—a world which yields him no true self-consciousness, but only lets him see himself through the eyes of others, of measuring one's souls, two thoughts, two unreconciled strivings; two warring ideals in one dark body, whose dogged strength alone keeps it from being torn asunder. (Du Bois, 1903, 16, 17)

HISTORICAL CONTEXT

1619	Slaves arrive in America from Africa.
1861–1865	Civil War.
1863	Emancipation Proclamation.
1865–1877	Reconstruction period. Ku Klux Klan begins.
1903	Du Bois writes *The Souls of Black Folk.*
1909	NAACP founded.
1910–1920	Black migrations, south to north.
1914–1918	World War I.
1915	Knights of Ku Klux Klan reorganized.
1919	"Red summer," black war veterans and others are victimized.
1929–1936	Great Depression.
1939	Marian Anderson, denied Constitution Hall, sings before 75,000 at Lincoln Memorial.
1939–1945	World War II.
1954	School segregation declared unconstitutional.
1955	Nonviolent bus boycott in Montgomery, Alabama .
1964	Martin Luther King is assassinated.
1964–1965	Civil rights legislation is passed.
1977	Louis Farrakan becomes head of Nation of Islam.
1984	Jessie Jackson founds Rainbow Coalition.
1995	California votes to cease affirmative action in state-supported universities.
1997	Schools in Oakland, California incorporate Ebonics into the curriculum creating nationwide controversy.
1997	Some southern black churches are destroyed by arson.
1998	Battles over affirmative action continue nationwide.

Case Examples

Sadie James, a Middle-Class African-American With Medical Problems But Good Family Support

Sadie James was born in rural Tennessee in 1925. Her ancestors were slaves and—later—sharecroppers and dirt farmers. When she was 5, her parents, with their five children, left the farm and moved to Memphis, where the father did factory work and the mother kept house for a rich white family. The children spent summers with their grandparents. Sadie married Ben James, a fellow high school graduate, before he joined the armed forces during World War II. After the war, he became a railroad porter. The Jameses had three daughters.

At first, Sadie and Ben James had few racial problems because African-Americans "knew their place." But their children went from segregated to integrated schools and from "colored-only" to "legal but not sanctioned" public places; and there was much turmoil during the civil rights era. The Jameses went on marches and sit-ins; some of their friends were jailed; one was killed. Eager to improve the lives of their daughters and to escape racial conflict, they moved to Oakland, California, when they heard that railroad jobs were available there. Mrs. James's brittle diabetes kept her unemployed, but she was active in the Baptist church and as a devoted mother.

The Jameses' daughter Joan became a nurse, and their daughter Helen became a teacher. Both married well, had children, and lived close by. Their third daughter, Cassie, a college dropout, divorced after having had three children and went back to college. Mr. and Mrs. James agreed to take care of her children, ages 8, 5, and 2.

In 1985, Ben James threatened the life of a workman who had done a poor, overpriced, plumbing job in their home. He was arrested, hospitalized, and medicated for paranoia. Two years later, he committed suicide. Sadie James, despite her grief, continued to care for her grandchildren; but soon afterward she suffered a stroke. She was placed in a skilled nursing facility for rehabilitation. When she wanted to go home, her physician agreed—if she could improve her ADLs. She worked diligently and was discharged. A gutsy woman, she tied her medications to her cane; and even though she had severe arthritis she regained her driver's license.

One day, her daughter Joan noticed a jar of lemon water in the refrigerator. Mrs. James said it was for high blood pressure—a substitute for costly medications. She also stopped taking insulin, and she ate high-fat southern cooking. Her relatives in Tennessee always took home remedies, she said. Her daughter was angry and upset but could not discuss her concerns: "I'm still her child," she told herself. However, she called Mrs. James's physician, who sent a VNA nurse to regulate the medications. Mrs. James then went through several nurses before she found one who was acceptable. This nurse was a black VNA who not only monitored the medications but also helped with practical issues and offered comfort. Throughout these trying times, Mrs. James's daughters never confronted her about her noncompliance, although they were worried. "She's our mother, and we must obey *her*," they said.

Otis Brown, an African-American From an Impoverished Environment With Depression and No Family Support

Otis Brown was born in 1925 in Arkansas, the second of Harley and Mary Brown's seven children. His grandparents were freed slaves who became sharecroppers during the Reconstruction period. His parents persisted in sharecropping despite poverty and prejudice in the postwar, Jim Crow south.

As a boy, Otis Brown worked the fields, so he attended his one-room segregated school only during nonfarming months. He went no further than third grade. Owing to inadequate health services, three of his siblings died of dysentery, but he himself was healthy. Aware of lynchings and the general misfortunes of young Negro men, he had a pervasive sense of danger and anxiety and was always on guard with whites. As an adult, he formed few intimate relationships, and because of his poverty, he postponed marriage.

Mr. Brown was drafted during World War II and later honorably discharged, but he was frightened because he knew about the Red Summer following World War I. He migrated to Milwaukee, got a job in a foundry, and married Mattie Hoover. They had two children, Marcella and Matthew. They lived happily in a segregated but nice neighborhood until Matt was killed by a drunk driver. Mattie became ill, and she too died—of inadequate medical care, her husband believed.

Depressed about Mattie's death, Mr. Brown ignored Marcella who felt abandoned and eventually moved back to the south, with the help of her minister. Mr. Brown, angry, cut off contact with the church, abused alcohol, and limped through life. In 1971, he moved in with Annie Markham, but she soon left him because he was too strict and nasty to her three children.

That year, Mr. Brown's foundry declared bankruptcy, and he lost his job—as a result of the company's mismanagement, he also lost his pension. Again depressed, penniless, and now hearing-impaired, he was physically and emotionally exhausted by his personal problems and by his years of heavy, dirty, noisy, foundry work. After treatment in an ER, he was referred to the local VA hospital, where he was incorrectly diagnosed as schizophrenic with paranoid features. An antipsychotic medication worsened his condition. Later, his diagnosis was changed to major depression and he was given Elavil. But, back home, still distrustful of the medical establishment, he discontinued his medication.

For the following decade, he received Veterans' benefits, SSI, and Social Security that paid for a two-room apartment in a low-income, high-crime area. He saw friends at the local pool parlor. An older friend, Betty Smith, looked in on him. When his arthritic condition worsened, though, he withdrew from those contacts. Ms. Smith then called the Milwaukee Department of Aging. This case study will be continued in Chapter 11.

Enid Maxwell, a Working-Class Caribbean Black Woman With Minimal Family Support

Enid Maxwell was born in Nassau, British West Indies, in 1905, the fifth child of merchant parents. She completed elementary school with excellent sewing and language skills. In 1927, she emigrated to London, where she worked as a seamstress. A son, Daniel, was born. She also had a daughter, who died.

After World War II, Ms. Maxwell immigrated to Brooklyn and did dressmaking there. She scrimped but was not able to save much. However, her union had a small pension fund. Her son Daniel finished junior college and became a bookkeeper and an unpaid minister. At intake, he was divorced and living in Queens. He had three adult children but saw them infrequently. Ms. Maxwell, a loner, had no church connections; her son was her only "support person," but they were not close. When she retired, she moved into public housing and enjoyed events at a "Neighborhood House" where she was well liked, being a soft-spoken lady. She did arts and crafts and helped with a the Sunshine Club for shut-ins. But her own health began to fail.

At age 72, she was diagnosed with Parkinson's disease, and some dementia appeared. Her son did her finances, and a Human Resources case manager arranged for home care. But her disease progressed rapidly, and she soon required full-time (12–12) home care. She gave up sewing and her activities at the center, but her aide wheeled her there for lunch in good weather. Soon her symptoms were severe; her short-term memory was gone, she fell often, and she was refusing medication. ("It burns up my stomach and brings back my old cancer," she said.). Concurrently, governmental cutbacks led to a review of her "12–12" status.

Daniel Maxwell was told that a nursing home, less expensive than 12–12, would be recommended. He was incensed, saying she would deteriorate even further there. He preferred sending her back to her sister in Nassau, where she would be happier. An alternative was a "sleep-in." But the staff thought that this, and Daniel's plan, would be too risky. The only way 12–12 could continue would be to prove that Enid would deteriorate in a nursing home. "But she has already deteriorated," the staff said; "she is not oriented to either time or place and is a constant danger to herself."

Then some miracles happened. Daniel Maxwell returned from checking out Nassau as a resource and reported that it would not work. Just then, Ms. Maxwell's condition showed some improvement. Also, the center started to offer day treatment for frail elderly people that would give more support and integrate and mainstream some activities. A volunteer "buddy" would be provided for each "guest". The center would try Mrs. Maxwell.

Daniel Maxwell began counseling with Marie S., a staff member, to prepare him for possible nursing home placement. He had a need to be in charge and never to be proved wrong and thus was hard to work with. But Ms. S. praised him for being so concerned about his mother and for checking out Nassau—who knows? It might have worked. He began to visit some nursing homes, "just in case."

A Group of Black Elders With Problems of Substance Abuse

Henry Evans, An African-American From an Impoverished Environment, With Alcohol Dependence and Minimal Support

Henry Evans, age 57, was born in Florida. He was passed through fourth grade, but with a severe learning disability. At age 30, he moved to New York City to find work. His parents, by then deceased, had been laborers. He had a sister, but her whereabouts were unknown. He married in New York, but then left his wife; he telephones his only daughter no more than three times a year. However, a nephew from Florida, Jake Evans, visits often. While he was still in Florida, Henry Evans took mechanics courses at a vocational school and worked on and off in factories. He now works part-time doing minor mechanical jobs.

Mr. Evans started drinking early—in fact, his was an alcoholic family. But he boasted he only drank; he never took drugs. He was a "binge drinker" and once drunk became out of control. Waking up after a blackout, he would find his pockets empty and would be accused of broken promises. "Then the cops took me to CARP detox," he said, "and if I knew it existed, I would have done it sooner. I was shaking, had a big head, no sleep, sick as a dog. My disease called for a drink but the nurses, staff, showed me love and how to stop. They said that if I stayed here, I'd get well; and they showed me I wasn't alone. They told me they had been there themselves. I was a happy drunk, never hurt anyone, but I was killing myself."

Henry Evans had both black and white sponsors and counselors. "It doesn't matter; God loves us all," he said. He now has a spiritual life. He likes helping youngsters in AA, telling them about the disease and the 12 steps. He remarked that "some folks would rather take a drink than medicine." He also said that he spent his life running but is now safe in domiciliary care.

Bill Roberts, an African-American From an Impoverished Environment, With Chemical Dependency and No Family Support

Bill Roberts was born in Georgia. He quit school during fifth grade to work on local farms. At age 15, he ran away to Florida. His substance abuse began early—at age 5. An ongoing victim of abuse by his father, he was rewarded with "booze" for stealing liquor. He learned to get high to overcome his fear of his father.

Mr. Roberts married and thereafter moved back and forth between Florida and Georgia. After years of abusing alcohol, he switched to snorting cocaine—when he had the money. In Florida, he snorted a lot, became homeless, and was eventually "acting like a vegetable," he said. After drinking transmission oil for a cheap high, he began hallucinating and was hospitalized. He was then referred to CARP for dependency treatment. "What almost cost me my life, saved it," he said, "Now I have HIV, and I need this shelter. My life is a total wreck."

Arnold Jefferson, an African-American From an Impoverished Environment With Chemical Dependency and Fictive Kin Support

Arnold Jefferson left school after the third grade. He became a migrant worker in Alabama and later joined the army. "I learned to drink. My people were all nondrinking farmers and only drank soda and coffee." But he was paid for his migrant work in credit lines that covered the previous week's alcohol. He married and had two sons, but at age 40, he left this family to do migrant work in Florida. There he lived in a rooming house with a new adopted "sister." Proudly, he said that he had sent money home until he was hospitalized for TB at age 62. After that, his new sister took care of him until he contacted pneumonia, entered a VA hospital, and then went to CARP for treatment of alcoholism. "By then, I knew the stuff made me sick and I had to stop fooling myself," he said.

Now, at age 74, Mr. Jefferson has been living at the CARP domiciliary since 1978. He is happy. He knows he cannot live outside, because he would drink again. He works as a gardener, goes to AA meetings, and believes that God brought him to CARP. He has twice-monthly passes to visit his sister, but there he must attend church, an AA meeting, and family dinner; he must return by Sunday night. He knows he needs CARP's strict rules and its counseling—which uses a concrete, repetitive approach, employment, and appropriate community resources. He is supported by Social Security, veterans' benefits, state and county funds, and his own minimal earnings. He believes that his "real family" is waiting for him in Georgia, where he left them, and he plans to return someday.

Marie Wilson, an Upper-Class Black Island Woman With Alcohol Dependence and Good Family Support

Marie Wilson's ancestors came to the Virgin Islands as slaves. When he was freed, her grandfather stayed on as the manager of a sugar plantation. Later generations were well-educated, hard-working, and they prospered. In fact, they became one of the island's leading black families, respected especially for helping to provide education and employment for island youngsters.

Mrs. Wilson's parents, both ministers, sent their children to Bible colleges on the mainland. It was on the mainland that she met and married her husband, William. They returned to the island, where William became a successful importer. Marie was a homemaker. She used her teacher-training to direct a Sunday school—and to raise three children who went on to high-ranking stateside universities and successful professional careers. While family and church were her main interests, her husband's business was also a paramount concern. She entertained graciously; she was articulate, well-informed, well-groomed and beautiful—a social asset to him.

In 1994, Mrs. Wilson's parents were killed in a plane crash. Church friends and family supported her in her grief; but after the funeral, her children returned to the states, and her husband was cold. A year later, a hurricane all but wiped out the island and Mrs. Wilson's home and church were destroyed. Her husband absented himself more, and she learned he was consoling—and in love with—another woman, who had also had losses from the hurricane.

Mrs. Wilson was devastated. Her physician prescribed Valium for her "nerves," but it did not always work. She began drinking rum to get through the night and, later, the day. She had never been a "drinker," and it did not take much—given her advancing age, her small size, her diabetes, and her use of Valium—to make her drunk. When she was rushed to an ER with diabetic complications, her children came home.

After detox and diabetic stabilization at an island hospital and an intervention by her children and physician, Mrs. Wilson was admitted to Hanley-Hazelden in Florida for its 28-day treatment of late-life alcoholism. Initially, she objected, denying that she had a problem; but she accepted the plan when her children promised to accompany her to Hanley-Hazelden. She vacillated between welcoming the prospect of being cared for and feeling terrible shame. She suffered from low self-esteem due to her husband's rejection and a self-concept damaged by her own "fallen behaviors."

In treatment, she was polite. But despite this, and despite her intelligence, she was only outwardly cooperative and did not accept her alcoholism as a disease. She clung to the issues of shame and chastised herself for sin and wrong-doing, believing that her parents, in heaven, were ashamed of her. Fearing a return to isolation and alcohol, a daughter suggested that Mrs. Wilson move in with her. But Mrs. Wilson was determined to rebuild her life— at home and in church—on the island. She agreed to follow through with aftercare, meetings, counseling, and a sponsor; and the staff helped to set them up. But back on the island, still ashamed, she did not respond to their outreach efforts.

Six months later, the Wilsons' marriage was formally dissolved. Mrs. Wilson voluntarily readmitted herself to Hanley-Hazelden, saying she could finally admit she was "powerless over alcohol and it was making her life unmanageable." Now, able to express her anger toward her husband, she was ready to work on her grief and shame—which had been an impediment to her treatment in the past. After completing inpatient work, she availed herself of ongoing treatment resources on her island and also returned to H-H regularly for aftercare. She is currently administrating an alcoholism prevention program for island youths and is an active AA volunteer.

Chapter 10

The AA Ethnic Lens

Du Bois's (1903) words, opening Part IV, are still relevant; they describe the struggle of African Americans for a merged identity in an alien world. A Harvard scholar and founder of the National Association for the Advancement of Colored People (NAACP), Du Bois is still honored as an eloquent black spokesperson.

Here, in accordance with current custom and the U.S. Census, we shall be using the terms black and African American (AA) to designate American people of black African ancestry. Other black Americans who came to the United States from Africa via the Caribbean Islands shall be so identified. But not all of your geroclients call themselves African American. At age 102, Bessie Delany (1993, p. 75) said,

> I don't use the word black very often to describe myself and my sister. To us, black was a person who was black, and honey, I mean *black as your shoe*. I'm not black, I'm brown. Actually, the best word to describe me, I think, is colored. I am a colored woman or a Negro woman. Either one is okay. People dislike those words now. Today they use *African American*. It wouldn't occur to me to use that. I prefer to think of myself as American, that's all.

If your geroclients prefer being called colored or Negro, be aware that younger members of their families may be offended by these terms. Some AA elders I asked said, as Delany did, "Just call me American." Just as not all elders are alike, not all African

American elders (AAs) are alike, and not all AA elders are like all of the younger AA cohorts. This is a very diverse population with many differences, and the reader is again warned not to stereotype. We shall be discussing general trends and contrasting them with intergroup differences, with other ethnic groups, and with the dominant culture, but that is only a starting point. It will be up to each gerocounselor to move from the general to the specific.

Demographics

African Americans are the largest ethnic category in the United States, and black elders are the fastest-growing segment of the total black population. Between 1970 and 1980, the numbers of elders increased 34 percent, compared with a 16 percent increase in the total black population. The 1990 census reported 2.5 million (8 percent) blacks over age 65; 230,000 (9 percent) of those were over 85. There are 63 black males for every 100 females over age 65. Among both white and black males and females, black females have the longest life expectancy. They will experience the most significant increase in the total elderly population (AARP, Minority Affairs, 1995).

Of the black population, 82 percent live in cities that are 50 percent or more black, and 59 percent live in the southeastern states. Of older AA elders, 20 percent live in extended families, compared to 12 percent of their white counterparts (Hooyman & Kiyak, 1996). Only 3–4 percent of nursing home patients in the United States are black; and of all those over 85, 8.4 of percent males and 13.5 percent of black females are institutionalized, compared with 15.8 percent of white males and 26.4 percent of white females (National Caucus and Center on Black Aged, 1987).

Many black elders live in poverty today, for several reasons. Racism has reduced opportunities for adequate health care, preventive care, education, and job training; and many low-paying jobs were not covered by Social Security and medical insurance. Because their life expectancy is lower, because few have private pensions, and because they tend to receive lower Social Security benefits, blacks also receive less retirement income than comparable whites. In 1988, 32 percent of the black elderly population was below the poverty level, compared to 10 percent of whites and 22 percent of Hispanic Americans. Also, the prevalence of chronic diseases, and hence disabilities, among blacks is twice as high as among whites, and many blacks are forced to retire earlier because of health problems (Richardson, 1990).

Immigration and Migration Experiences

African Americans—unlike most other immigrants—did not come to the United States to improve their lot in life. Instead, the ancestors of America's black elders were captured, purchased, and brought to American English colonies, beginning in 1619, to become plantation slaves. Later, many were born into slavery. For Afro-Caribbeans, immigration experiences were different. Coming to the United States from a society similar in history, language, and religion, and with technical and professional skills, they realized material advantages here, as Enid Maxwell and Marie Wilson's children did.

Most black slaves—descendants of hunters, gatherers, and farmers skilled in stonework—came from 25 nations south of the Sahara desert in West Africa. Most lived along Egyptian routes where traders disseminated goods and the Islamic religion. African-Muslim societies were dominant from the 12th to the 16th centuries.

A large African merchant class developed, trading slaves, gold, and ivory for cloth, tools, and weapons. The Portuguese established trading posts in the 1500s and were the first to export African slaves. Other Europeans soon followed suit. In 1619, Dutch traders sold 20 West Africans to colonists in Jamestown, Virginia; 425,000 were to follow. Over half of these American slaves—from what is now Angola and Nigeria—had tribal connections with the Ashanti, Bambara, Fulani, Ibo, Malenke, or Yoruba. Their cultures were mainly based on the extended family and religion.

The Civil War and emancipation are credited with ending American slavery as it was known, but a new type of slavery created by racism, poverty, and oppression then emerged. During the reconstruction period of the later 1800s, the Ku Klux Klan (KKK) was formed and Jim Crow, a legally sanctioned practice of inequality against blacks, began under the guise of "separate but equal." However, many black families were also reunited, marriages were legalized, a black graduated from West Point, and Booker T. Washington founded Tuskegee Institute.

In the early 1900s, over 500,000 blacks, mostly intact two-parent families, migrated from the south to the urban north in search of jobs and education. Du Bois wrote *The Souls of Black Folk* and founded the NAACP, and black art and music (jazz) were part of the "Harlem renaissance." Marcus Garvey preached racial pride in a "back to Africa" political-labor movement that amassed over 1 million black followers.

But Otis Brown was anxious as the KKK also grew to over 5 million members, lynchings continued, and then, despite the fact that over 100,000 blacks had fought in World War I, their victorious homecoming was overshadowed by the "red summer" of 1919, when riotous violence occurred against black GIs and others in some major cities.

The 1930s brought some progress. The Great Depression caused increased poverty among northern urban blacks, southern share-croppers, and whites alike; but it also brought integration into the labor movements (1935) and more AAs into government. Blacks took pride in Jessie Owens's Olympic victory and Marian Anderson's concert at the Lincoln Memorial before 75,000 people, after she had been turned away from Constitution Hall.

Although racial discrimination was banned in national defense contracts, troops were still segregated in World War II and remained so until 1948. Black soldiers returned to a civilian life that included segregated businesses and facilities (drinking fountains, etc.), poll taxes, and antimiscegenation laws in the south. But discrimination was not just in the south. In the early 1950s, I lived in a town in central Illinois where "Negroes" were forbidden on the streets after sundown. Soon afterward, in northern Illinois, I could not legally eat at a diner with a black friend.

The civil rights era of the 1950s and beyond helped to push back some inequities. The Supreme Court had supposedly ended school segregation in 1954 (*Brown v. Board of Education*), but peaceful marches and boycotts led by Martin Luther King, Jr., and others were often met with violence. Sadie and Ben James watched their friends jailed—and one killed—as they participated in nonviolent sit-ins and marches. In 1961 Affirmative Action began and King's assassination in 1964 resulted in the passage of the Civil Rights Act of 1965 which integrated schools and public facilities. But anger, among both blacks and whites, also mounted—resulting in conflicts and a backlash.

Since those tumultuous times, blacks have continued to gain power, but their vast intracategory differences have not always produced a united front. These differences range from the ideas of Louis Farrakan, who became head of the Nation of Islam in 1977, to Jessie Jackson's, who founded the Rainbow Coalition in 1984, to Colin Powell's—Powell, a declared Republican, could have been the presidential candidate for either party in 1996.

Most black elders, such as Sadie and Ben James and Otis Brown, learned about slavery at their grandparents' knees and lived through the history sketched above. Theirs is a saga of hardship and discrimination in a racist society, and different cohorts dealt with it in various ways.

Today's AA elders, sometimes called "Martin Luther King blacks", are not always in agreement with younger, more militant AAs. These elders, such as Sadie James, are sometimes berated by their children for having adopted a melting-pot model and assimilating into a white society that denied them their roots, their pride, and their sense of unique identity.

Cultural Values

African American culture is defined as bicultural, and AA children are socialized to assimilate into both the white and the Afro culture. At home, standards of child rearing, language, communication, religion, and family composition sometimes differ from those of the dominant society. Parents are caring, but discipline can have a harsh, toughening-up quality, in preparation for survival in a hostile, racist environment. That was how Otis Brown was raised; but his live-in girlfriend left him for being too harsh with her children. AA parents raise sons to be both assertive and acquiescent and to confront when necessary (Locke, 1992, p. 22).

In a classic example of blaming the victim, blacks are criticized for a culture of poverty and female-centered families. Social reformers focus on welfare mothers but forget highly successful, educated, wealthy, and political blacks like Marie Wilson. Defenders of blacks stress that when AAs differ from the dominant culture, that does not necessarily reflect their inability to assimilate but, rather, reflects remnants of an African society and subsequent deprivation. When blacks achieve middle-class status in the dominant culture, they often feel tugs from both their new status and the lower rungs of the class system they left behind (Devore & Schlesinger, 1991).

Much has been written about the gender roles of African Americans and the "absent male" in the black family. In Africa, blacks enjoyed a culture that included a strong but complicated family life based on a lineage system. Marriages, linked to religion as well as political and economic lines between villages, were highly ritualized events that set up male-governed family groups.

The idea that black slaves were passive, acquiescent and deficient in family and culture myths, is a discounted by modern historians (Haley, 1976). Although slaveowners tried to diminish black family life, small nuclear families existed in the United States. The few who did survive to old age lived in extended families. Owing to the selling and relocation of their members, these families had no autonomy, little time for children, and little or no stability. But as early as the 1700s, blacks struggled to maintain extended family networks and, when possible, developed fictive kin, strong sibling loyalties, intergenerational ties, and unique naming practices.

Some linguists believe that African Americans experienced deficient language development in early childhood that resulted in inadequate communication skills in standard English. Others contend that AAs use a well-structured, highly developed black English system rooted in pidgin, Creole, and certain West African linguistic rules.

African American arts also have unique characteristics. Hale-Benson (1982) described them as circular, episodic arrangements of small, short units leading to ongoing, open-ended mini-climaxes.

Cuisine includes African, Caribbean, soul food from the slave kitchens, and today's AA cooks. Peppers give African foods their distinctive flavor, and a favorite concoction is a tomato-based stew, palava, made of spicy beef and spinach and served over rice. In the Caribbean, the stewpot is never emptied; peppers and juices of the cassava root are added as the pot gets depleted, and French, Spanish, English, and Indian cookery are melded with African and West Indian spices.

The genius of the slave kitchens was the ability to transform meats of poor quality into delicious meals with abundant vegetables and even weeds. Tripe, fried squirrel, pig's feet, ham hocks, and neckbones were popular, as were wild greens, onions, corn-meal, beans, and sweet potato pie. Additional foods included, "short'ning" bread, fried biscuits, hushpuppies, hoecakes, crackling cornbread, and redeye gravy.

Soul food, still favored by poor and rural elders, is cooked in an abundance of lard and is high in fat, cholesterol, and sodium, thus contributing to high rates of heart disease, high blood pressure, and diabetes.

AAs celebrate two unique holidays, Juneteenth and Kwanzaa. Juneteenth, a celebration of the reading of the Emancipation Proclamation in Texas in 1865, might include a menu of jerk pork, pasta vegetable salad, pickled beets, red rice, oven-roasted potatoes, and toasted butter pecan cake. Kwanzaa lasts seven days, from December 26 to January 1, to focus on seven principles (called *Nguzo Saba*) to be learned and acted upon all year: (1) unity, (2) self-determination, (3) collective work and responsibility, (4) cooperative economics, (5) purpose, (6) creativity, and (7) faith. A Kwanzaa celebration might include blessing soup (chicken), sweet and sour cabbage, kale with tomatoes and onions, rice primavera, and walnut sweet potato pie (Medearis, 1994).

Suffering and surviving have been two major conditions of AA peoples, and today, problems continue to plague the black late-life family. The prevalence of chronic disease (as seen in all of our case examples) and hence disability is twice as high among AA elders as among whites; many AAs, as already noted, are forced to retire earlier because of poor health. But while blacks' life expectancies are similar to or slightly lower than those of whites in the dominant culture, there is a remarkable occurrence called the crossover effect. "After age 75, life expectancy [for blacks] is actually greater than for whites, due to a combination of biological vigor, psychological strength, and resources for coping with stress, such as religious practices that link individuals to the community" (Hooyman & Kiyak, 1996, p. 444).

Another evidence of blacks' survival skills is seen in caregiving. The family, particularly the elder female, is often the caregiver for the sick, partly because nursing homes are considered unacceptable to many for AA long-term care. And AA caregivers report less stress than white caregivers. Because her employed daughters could not quit their jobs, Sadie James entered a nursing home—but she entered it reluctantly and worked doggedly for discharge.

Reports of high life satisfaction among AA elders are linked to the strong values of intergenerational interdependence in the black family, to a culture that sponsors a strong support system among friends and fictive kin, and to spiritual and other resources derived from black churches. Participation in religion—Christian and Muslim—is high among AA elders and provides companionship, encouragement, and financial and emotional support as well as spiritual benefits. The losses experienced by Otis Brown when his anger forced him out of the church and by Marie Wilson when her despondency and alcoholism moved her away were enormous— and this was at a time when they most needed such a resource.

In sum, the life of the average black elder appears to be socially and positively integrated despite economic hardships, chronic diseases, and early aging problems. It is important too to remember that "African-American culture [today] is an expression of the desire of African Americans to decide their own destiny through control of their own political organizations and the establishment and preservation of their cultural, economic, and social institutions" (Locke, 1992, p. 27). However, neither their success in aging nor their self-determination should be used by the dominant society as an excuse for relinquishing its responsibility to provide programs for those in need, such as the poor elderly.

Issues: Sources of Pain and Pride

Years of racism and poverty led to conditions that earned AAs a "disadvantaged status." Participants in the Million Man March of 1995 called attention to grim statistics about higher rates of prison admissions (42 percent in prisons), unemployment (twice that of whites), homicide (the leading cause of deaths for AAs), juvenile delinquency, female alcoholism, poverty (34 percent are below the poverty level compared with 11.55 percent of whites), and school dropouts. Sue and Sue (1990) noted that many of the same people are counted several times.

Many AAs receive less pension income than whites, and because of their lower life expectancies they do not get the same benefits as whites in terms of years. In 1988, 32 percent of black elders were below the poverty level, compared with 10 percent of whites and 22 percent of Hispanics. Many black elders mourn the loss of offspring in Vietnam or to the illegal drug culture. "Today some may find themselves rearing grandchildren and great-grandchildren because their children are substance abusers who are unable to care for their offspring" (Richardson, 1990, p. 3).

Black elders have good and bad memories. Strides were made during the civil rights era, but some say this only drove racism underground and it is alive and healthy today. Still, progress has been made, and to many elders the contrasts are striking.

Black schoolchildren now learn not only about Booker T. Washington and W. E. B. Du Bois, but also about a host of others who were once slaves or progeny of slaves. Examples include the civil rights activists David Walker, George Bush, Frederick Douglas, Sojourner Truth, Whitney Young, and Martin Luther King, Jr.; the governmental figures Robert Small, Robert Brown Elliott, Blanche K. Bruce, Robert Weaver, Mary McCleod Bethune, Andrew Young, Thurgood Marshall, Adam Clayton Powell; the prominent inventors Jan Matzeliger and Granville Woods; the guide and explorer, Benjamin Banneker; the surveyors Matthew Henson and James Beckwourth; the scientists Daniel Hale Williams, Charles Drew, and James Dumpson; the journalists David Walker and Ida B. Wells; the business leaders Charles Clinton Spaulding and A.G. Gaston; and social workers such as Thelma L. Eaton. Jean-Baptiste Pointe du Sable, a Haitian fur trader, erected the first house in Chicago.

Blacks have been well represented in the arts by poets such as Phyllis Wheat and Maya Angelou and writers such as William Holmes Borders, W. E. B. Du Bois, Malcom X, James Baldwin, Toni Morrison, and Sarah and Elizabeth Delany. The musicians, actors, and athletes who have also added to this rich tapestry of American culture are too numerous to mention.

Many black elders proudly hope that their grandchildren will learn about slavery and its destructive consequences, the enormous strengths and resilience that it took to endure those years, and the courageous long-time civil rights efforts that began long before the dramatic 1960s. When one writes about the need to focus on strengths in gerocounseling, it is not hard to find those qualities in most black elders today. They have truly overcome.

EXERCISE

Think about the AA elders described at the beginning of this section and other black elders that you know. How could any of the historical events listed at the beginning of this chapter have affected their lives, their current problems, or the problems of their cohorts? Consider the dimensions of the Ethnic Lens: identity, demographics, immigration and migration experiences, cultural values, and special issues. What part might any of them play in their present problems, beliefs, and attitudes?

Chapter 11

The AA Gero Chi Lens

Again, let us adjust the Gero Chi Model; this time we will view it through the AA Ethnic Lens. Immediately we must alter the *self-system,* because the independent self of the dominant white society changes to a dual, interdependent self in a flexible, black family system.

The Self-System

Self Concept

Much has been written about the struggle of the black self to maintain a bicultural balance between two almost antithetic worlds. As early as 1903, Du Bois wrote,

> From this must arise a painful self-consciousness, an almost morbid sense of personality and a moral hesitancy which is fatal to self-confidence. . . . Such a double life, with double thoughts, double duties, and double social classes, must give rise to double words, and double ideals. (1961, pp. 148–149)

Back in 1972, Barnes doubted that the black child could develop a positive self-concept in the closed European American system. Early learning about the undesirability of black skin resulted in an incomplete self-image, a rejection of one's own group, or a negative self-image and a preference for whites. Each reaction can have negative effects on one's cognitive and affective status and orientation toward achievement.

Valentine (1971) described a bicultural model that differentiated the African American self from the European American self; and the Afrocentric theory of Baldwin (1984) held that African self-extension and self-consciousness were basic to a positive black identity.

Powell (1983) found little evidence of real self-hatred or flat racial identification among AAs. There was some "dissonance in the self," but not enough to produce strong group rejection or shame (p. 59). The black child developed a good sense of self despite the pervasive destructive impact of racism; but the self, she wrote, was a collective self, composed of many facets.

One would think that the self-esteem profile of today's black elders, marred by numerous discontinuities, adversities, and insults, would include negative self-attitudes; but paradoxically, these black elders, usually highly respected in their families and churches, have developed positive self-esteem from these close informal contacts.

Gender

Edmonds (1994) expanded the paradox to black females' perception of their health. Many, despite social, economic—and health—problems, tend to perceive their health as better than it is. This seems to be due to unique survival mechanisms, ways of handling stress and utilizing resources that enhance self-esteem, such as family and spirituality. The longer a black woman lives, the more satisfied she becomes with her health. Black elder women are less likely to commit suicide than whites, for example.

Much has been written about the strong position of the black grandmother in AA matriarchies. But notice is also taken of her vulnerable position, her quadruple jeopardy: being old, black, poor, and female (Jackson, 1975).

Battered AA women use informal support systems to cope with domestic violence. Thus much battering goes unreported, with the result that rates for AAs appear lower than rates for comparable whites. AA women usually view battering as the black man's displaced anger and aggression in response to racism.

The black male's role varies among families and individuals. The stereotype of the absent black husband, father, or adult son is considered an exaggeration by many, who argue that AA males, functioning as providers and role models, are present in over half of AA families, and that older men are more likely to be successful providers than younger men. Wilson (1987) conducted a study in inner-city Chicago and reported that most unemployed black men preferred mainstream work and family patterns, but a lack of job and career opportunities prevented them from contributing to their families and relating to successful black men or to society. Black communities recognize males for valued qualities—friendship, compassion, sharing, honesty, courage, and self-control—more than for providing material goods (Daly, Jennings, Beckett, & Leashore, 1995, p. 242).

But statistics are alarming. Family and neighborhood violence is a major problem in depressed black areas. AA men have a suicide rate four times higher than AA women, and their rates of homicide and incarceration are also alarmingly high. Affirmative Action, an attempt (since 1961) to rectify other problems, has received mixed evaluations in this area. Sometimes black males are placed unfairly in competition for education and job opportunities with black women, creating additional family stress.

Spirituality

A high degree of involvement in religion is seen among the black elderly. For some, religion is linked to faith healing. Most blacks are Christian (mostly Baptist and Methodist) but the Nation of Islam, a black Muslim sect, is growing in numbers and visibility. Haitians practice Vodum, a blend of Roman Catholicism and African religion, called "root medicine."

Although religion has provided an emotional and psychological haven from a harsh and discriminatory social system, it has not been just a band-aid used to forestall necessary social action. It functions as a base for social action and reform; and it adds to personal and group identity, perceptions of personal control and efficacy, emotional well-being and mental health, the provision of social support, and being influential in the broader black community (Taylor & Chatters, 1991).

Edmonds (1994) lamented that religion has sometimes led to

dysfunctional coping, such as poor behaviors related to illness—notably medical noncompliance among black females. If Marie Wilson's ultimate goal is heaven and the path there is through suffering, then she may read the Bible and pray instead of seeking medical help or trying to solve her problem.

Psychosocial Tasks

Erikson's psychosocial tasks (1950) have been used to shed light on the personality development of black and other elders and also on intergenerational differences in child rearing that might cause family conflicts. The AA Ethnic Lens, of course, influences how these tasks are worked through. Otis Brown's continuing history is an example.

> Despite his pervasive depression, Otis Brown felt pride in being 80—he was proud of his independence, his self-sufficiency, and simply his survival, all achieved despite countess adversities. He may have been a "Negro man," looked down on by whites, but he was "a real man." From the days when he had been brought to the fields to suckle at his mother's breast, he knew he was special to his family. His religion had taught him that he was one of God's "special children" and that, if not here, rewards would come to him in heaven.
>
> Mr. Brown had been a hard worker in the fields as a boy, in school, in the army, in the foundry. He had earned his way, provided for his family, and helped when relatives needed money; he had shared with others. He believed that if one obeyed the commandments and worked hard enough, things would work out. He loved his parents, his relatives, his wife and his children, but they had all been taken away from him. If this was God's plan, he was angry at God.
>
> After age 80, Mr. Brown began to feel that life was near the end. His body ached, and he longed to join his wife, who had died. He was lost in reverie for the most part, and even food, hygiene, a clean, warm place, were not important anymore. A life review evoked bitterness and blame; it was that damn drunk driver's fault, the minister's fault, or the union's fault, or the fault of the landlord who turned off his heat. It was his girlfriend's fault for taking the kids' side. He knew that his few friends just laughed at him.
>
> This case study will be continued later.

Hope (Trust versus Mistrust)

Trust is established through nurturing and protection to ensure infants' survival. In most extended AA families, the infant has stable relationships with loving people, and receives enough attention to develop responsive accommodations to others.

Will (Autonomy versus Shame)

Here, one needs to develop appropriate ways to meet physical needs, gain control of impulses, and develop behaviors to protect against racism (Powell, 1983).

Purpose (Initiative versus Guilt)

Acquiring physical, mental, and social competence begins here. At age 3 or 4, black children become aware of racial differences and start to acquire a sexual identity believed to be created and reinforced through modeling by the same-sex parent or the most nurturing parent. One can only speculate what happens in some AA (and other) family systems when fathers are absent and mothers may reject male children.

However, in many black families with a single female parent, there are significant males in the extended family, or a fictive father figure is present, and many gender-shaping processes—not just the father as model—are operating. Fatherlessness does not seem to result in sex-identity confusion, but a model is lacking for the roles of husband and father to guide boys later in their own family lives (Wilson, 1987). Also, owing to the flexibility of AA families, male and female roles may not be clearly defined.

Competence (Industry versus Inferiority)

Here, the task is to learn about the physical and social environment and appropriate behaviors for given situations and people. Early on, the middle-class black child is encouraged to set goals that offer the greatest security. By age 7, AA children are aware that their racial group is devalued, regardless of where they live or the socioeconomic status of their families (Norton, 1983). The goal for inner-city black children is survival.

Fidelity (Identity versus Diffusion)

AA families meet the symbolic needs of their children that shape possible identities. The naming process—giving a child a special name with a symbolic meaning—is an example. Names may reflect an esteemed relative or a special virtue.

Love (Intimacy versus Isolation)

Autonomy without disrupting family ties is a major task as the young black adult creates family and work lives. One is expected to help later siblings coming along (as Otis Brown always did) and to reside close to the family.

Although family life and male authority were stressed in the ancestral African culture, the system of slavery tried to destroy the institutions of black marriage and family, thus making long-term commitments difficult.

Care (Generativity versus Stagnation)

Here, one learns to balance individual and group goals. Black extended kinship networks aid in family survival by fostering interdependence and providing help to members of all ages. Elders are supported by collective efforts.

The role of the black husband and father varies. Usually, the black father, as provider, regardless of income, is recognized as head of the household although this role is often weakened by job and money constraints. In the flexible black family, roles may be reversed, with an unemployed father providing child care while the mother goes out to work.

Wisdom (Integrity versus Despair)

Sometimes this psychosocial stage goes awry for a black person. In Otis's story, for example, negative past memories remained. When an elder's adult child has HIV or is addicted to drugs or alcohol, the elder may mourn a lost dream for the next generation. If an elder is unable to assume care of grandchildren because of illness or disability, despair can take hold—unless late-life expectations and roles are revised. This is a task aided by faith, religious beliefs, and family values (Baker, 1991).

However, most black elders report a high degree of life satisfaction as regards basic physiological and symbolic needs. This requires a sense of reality; a coherent world; a belief system; and a sense of self-esteem, personal control, and social affiliation. It also depends on having lifelong resources and finding a balance between personal strength and vulnerability. The internal integrity achieved by the majority of black elders at this last stage helps them to relate to and manage their external world.

THE SUBSET SYSTEMS

The AA Ethnic Lens continues to entail adaptations to the AA Gero Chi Model as we view its biopsychosocial systems.

The Biological System

Health Status

Blacks have a life expectancy of 69.6 years, compared with 75.2 years for nonminorities; but once a black reaches age 70, a crossover effect occurs, and the life expectancy for AAs becomes higher than that for whites. The leading causes of deaths among AA elderly people are cancer, heart disease, stroke, diabetes, and cirrhosis of the liver. Black men have 25 percent higher incidence of cancer than whites, with more cancers of the lung, prostate, stomach, and pancreas. Deaths from cirrhosis of the liver among blacks are double those among whites; and deaths from esophageal disorders are ten times higher. One in three blacks has hypertension. Twice as many black men die from stroke as white men, and their death from stroke rate is more than double that of other minorities. Blacks also are at higher risk than whites for diabetes (57 percent higher for black men; 100 percent higher for black women), and complications often follow. Up to age 74, as a group, blacks exceed standards for healthy weight and body fat; 80 percent of the diabetes in black women is attributed to obesity (AARP, 1990b, p. 2.).

Health Maintenance

Diet, environment, lifestyle, and heredity all play a role in the health of all age groups in all races. Improper diet (salted, smoked, and pickled foods) is considered a big factor in 35 percent of deaths from cancer among AAs. More blacks than whites smoke (fewer cigarettes but brands with higher tar); obesity and poverty are also linked to cancer.

While whites and most blacks tend to have similar dietary patterns, some differences exist. Blacks appear to consume fewer calories per day; black females age 55 to 64 report the lowest caloric intake. Social factors such as religion, geography, and income influence blacks' food choices. Older blacks, particularly those who are poorer and those with poor oral health, are more likely to skip meals and have less caloric intake.

Health-Related Beliefs and Practices

Many low-income blacks delay seeking medical help, ignore prevention, and use the emergency room for medical care. It is believed that black elders use long-term care facilities less because of costs, family patterns, discrimination, and a distrust of white institutions. But the lower number of AAs in nursing homes may also mean that black adults over 75 are more physically able than their white counterparts and that the flexible extended black family is offering more support to frail elders. Foster home care has been considered as an alternative for frail AA older persons without support.

Distrust of white institutions causes some AA elders to inadvertently sabotage their own medical care. Many have learned to falsify information and give only expected answers rather than relevant facts (Richardson, 1990).

Black folk medicine, a necessary accommodation to poverty and slavery, has roots in West Africa, the rural United States, Caribbean islands, and Judeo-Christian fundamentalism. One seeks help from a person who is considered most competent by those consulted, usually a "granny" or "old lady"—an older woman, versed in herbs, home remedies, and other folk healing, who treats ills with over-the-counter drugs such as baking soda, Epsom salts, garlic, herbs, and roots.

Traditional black elders perceive illness as related to good and evil, natural and unnatural; but many other older blacks seek mainstream medical care just as whites do. Different health beliefs and behaviors are often associated with age, cohort, level of education, urban versus rural residence, sex, and occupation (Richardson, 1990).

To more superstitious older blacks, unnatural illness (that which hangs on too long) may still be seen as a disharmony with nature caused by breaking a taboo, neglecting certain rites, or falling under the evil influence of another person (a witchcraft hex) and thus as lying outside the realm of modern medicine. All illness is considered curable by some elders, and chronicity is not recognized. A natural illness is caused by improper self-care (ingesting impurities, exposure to cold, inappropriate diet, etc.) and thin blood (the young and the old are believed to be more susceptible to illness because of thinner blood). Often such treatment is combined with a medical regimen, to the detriment of the latter and the patient's compliance.

Natural or unnatural, illness is sometimes perceived as a trial to be overcome through prayer and religious faith with the use of folk remedies or the help of modern biomedical technologies or both. Black community pharmacists play an important role by translating physician's prescriptions into folk concepts but may also carry and recommend patent medicines (Lydia Pinkham's Vegetable Compound, Humphrey's 11, and Black Draught) and drug ingredients such as turpentine, sulphur, asafetida, and camphor. Sadie James substituted lemon water for her medicines.

The Psychological System

AA elders may sometimes be less receptive than their adult children to today's concepts of mental health. The black family tended to provide psychiatric care until the desegregation of state hospitals, and blacks seldom received psychotherapy.

Racism existed in the mental health community, as elsewhere, and mental health professionals often practiced with apparent biases. In the early 1900s, blacks were believed to have more psychoses than whites but were also seen as happy and carefree, lacking the psychic framework to experience loss and depression.

Compared with whites, black adults in state hospitals were more likely to be diagnosed as schizophrenic and less likely to be diagnosed as alcoholic or depressed—despite the fact that alcohol abuse is likely among male elders and alcoholic hallucinations can resemble psychosis if not assessed carefully. Similarly, black manic-depressive patients in state hospitals were more likely than comparable whites to be diagnosed as schizophrenic. Such diagnoses have implications for prognosis, treatment, rehabilitation, and future employment opportunities. Sadie James's family believes that a failure to diagnose depression was probably a cause of Ben James's suicide.

Cognitive disorders are found similarly in all races and ethnic groups. While the reported prevalence of dementia is the same for blacks and whites (5–10 percent of the population), the actual prevalence may be higher for blacks—although this has not been documented (Richardson, 1990). Various racial groups have different patterns of dementing illnesses, depending on diet, environment, and heredity. For example, black women may have higher rates of multi-infarct dementia due to more obesity and hypertension. "Based on the medical problems of the black community which national studies have identified, the potential for an increased prevalence of head trauma, particularly in the African American males, may result in a high prevalence of clinically diagnosed Alzheimer's disease" (Baker, 1991, p. 7). Alcoholic dementia may also occur among younger blacks who reach the health care system at later stages.

Statistics about depression among black elders are lacking, but some studies show a higher prevalence of depressive illness (25 percent) among all medical populations relative to community-resident elders. As AAs reach their thirties and forties, their chance of developing chronic illnesses is higher than for other groups, so it may be safe to say that AA elders with active medical problems have a greater risk of depression. (Baker, 1991).

A healthy aspect of the AA culture has been its ability to retain a sense of peoplehood, pride in "blackness," and psychic security against all odds. Group identity plays a large role in the attainment of ego strength and self-esteem among AAs, and the group and family provide a buffer from outer assaults. Methods of survival such as respect for elders, sharing material needs and resources, and caring for one another—are learned in the family and group.

In sum, many AA elders, despite a lifetime of racism, poverty, and poor health, report more life satisfaction, happiness, and social integration than whites in better circumstances. This has been attributed to AAs' high levels of family support, participation in religion, and spiritual orientation (Hooyman & Kiyak, 1996).

The Sociological System

The AA Ethnic Lens dispels some myths about black families—the mistaken notion that they (1) are dysfunctional, (2) lack traditional values, (3) lack a father, (4) are female-dominated, and (5) perpetuate an unmotivated, nonproductive welfare-based lifestyle. Let us address these myths briefly.

Myth One

Are black families dysfunctional? A functional family is one that works and survives through its ups and downs. As slaves, AA families made valiant efforts to reunite. When that was impossible, they envisioned a reunion in the afterlife. Today, confronting the slavery of drugs and racism, families continue to serve as mutual support systems, and kinship bonds (fictive and real) help AAs to cope with problems. Boundaries are elastic, as a means of adaptation, and the fluid black family system is indeed functional.

Myth Two

Does the black family lack 'traditional values"? Whose values? Many AA family values predate those of the white majority, but the basic family models are dissimilar. The European family model is nuclear and stresses conjugality; the African family model is extended and stresses consanguinity. Both stress religion, education, and work. After slavery, the extended family became the focus—as in Africa, where blood kinship took precedence.

Myth Three

Does the black family tend to lack a father? As already noted, over half of black fathers surveyed are regarded as head of the household; and if fathers are not gainfully employed, parental roles are reversed. When a biologic father is not in residence, do not assume that he is psychologically absent: He may still be exerting influence on the family. Also, other family males may be functioning in the role of father for the children (Daly et al., 1995).

Myth Four

Is the black family female-dominated? In most AA families, the male is considered the head of the household regardless of the income he provides. But even in families headed by males, among many lower-class or rural southern blacks, consanquinity resulted in labeling the family matriarchical or female-headed.

While AA females often assume more family responsibilities than white women, that does not imply dominance. AA couples are sometimes more egalitarian than whites as regards sharing work. Often both work outside the home, and child care is delegated to an older sibling or grandparent—again, this is evidence of a flexible family system (Hines & Boyd-Franklin, 1982).

Myth Five

Does the black family perpetuate a nonproductive welfare-based lifestyle? Despite being undermined by a racist system, work and education rank high in most black families, as is seen in the growing number of blacks who study beyond the compulsory age and go on to higher education. Elders encourage children to take advantage of the opportunities now open to them.

Late-Life Marriages

Discord between black males and females is dealt with indirectly rather than through confrontation. Solutions, when sought, are informal. Separations are frequent; divorces are unusual. Even troubled marriages are usually considered lifelong because of religious convictions and a tendency toward long-suffering acceptance. As already noted, when a male is abusive, his partner may remain with him out of empathy.

Caregiving

Three out of five black elders are women, many of whom live in three-generation households where they care for and support grandchildren.

As with whites, the black family is the primary caregiving institution; but while filial responsibility and an interdependent extended-family system remain the norm, this is declining (Richardson, 1990). Probably because of economics more than race, AA elders are believed to be entitled to care by the family, having provided for their own offspring. Some observers attribute this tendency to the fluid "dependent-interdependent" nature of the AA family: each member provides help and receives help as needed. But some poor black families with very low incomes find the burden of caregiving impossible; others, who have fallen into drugs and crime, are not available.

The average age of elder AA caregivers is 55.8 (compared with whites' average age of 62). They are more likely than whites to be adult children or spouses, to get more help from family and friends, and to report feeling less burdened (Young, Kahana, & Waller, 1988).

Death and Dying

Practices of AAs regarding death and dying are similar to those of their white religious counterparts. Many blend Christian and Muslim religious practices with modified ceremonies that feature musical rhythms, patterns of speech, and rituals of worship from Africa. Funeral services vary. Some traditional Catholic and Episcopalians may grieve formally; Baptists and members of the Holiness Protestant Church are less formal, preferring lively hymns, obituary and poetry readings, and an emotional pastoral eulogy. At a Holiness ceremony, close relatives may shout or speak in tongues, rise with energy, and even jerk or move as a group to express grief; some people may faint. The body is viewed after the service before a burial (that is usually preferred over cremation). Haitians who practice Vodum believe that one must make peace with the collection of spirits around oneself at life events such as death.

Bereavement customs also vary. Older women may be more likely to follow traditional public mourning patterns, praying, wearing dark colors, and reducing activities. Cultural and individual differences determine the length of the bereavement period—from weeks to years. Ask each AA family about its specific beliefs and practices, as there are many differences (AARP, 1990).

Tasks of Aging

Aging tasks are similar for AAs and the general population. But like other minorities, AAs may find these tasks more difficult to achieve because of issues such as those noted in the Ethnic Lens. The task of independence must be altered to include the interdependence valued by African Americans.

As with other ethnic groups, we must add an additional task, the maintenance of continued harmony between the ethnic and the dominant cultures, so that one's final days can be spent in comfort, not despair. How much and whether one chooses or declines to acculturate or assimilate, is of course an individual decision.

> EXERCISE
>
> Think again of the case examples at the beginning of this section. After layering the Ethnic Lens onto the Gero Chi Model, what new information about AAs do you now have that adds to a greater understanding about these AA elders and their families and other black elders you know? What additional information do you need?

Chapter 12

AAs and Gerocounseling

Is gerocounseling with African Americans different from that with other categories? To find out, let us place the AA Ethnic Lens and the AA Gero Chi Lens on the Gerocounseling Model.

Generic Ethnogerocounseling of African Americans

This book has stressed that the basics of generic gerocounseling should apply to all cultures. But additionally, in ethnogerocounseling you are advised to first learn about the unique circumstances (including the culture) of each individual client and family, start where the client is, and let the client lead and show you the way. This is especially important in the AA category, where there are vast ethnic and class differences.

Ethics Skills

While most studies on ethics are medical, they have relevance for gerocounseling as well. The AA Ethnic Lens implies some surprising changes in the application of three ethical principles: autonomy, beneficence, and fidelity. It demonstrates that to be truly ethical, counseling must proceed individual by individual, family by family, culture by culture.

Autonomy

Many black clients, like Daniel Maxwell, will expect an egalitarian approach in which practitioner and client share in the decision-making process and the final determination is the client's. But many other traditional black elders—like Henry Evans, Bill Roberts, or Arnold Jefferson—may feel differently—wanting and needing a powerful helper to guide them in defining values and selecting appropriate interventions. Fewer nonwhites, for example, complete written advance directives than their white counterparts (Mouton, Johnson, & Cole, 1995).

Beneficence

Doing good extends beyond providing food, shelter, and medical care, although that is a good beginning with many poor minority clients—such as in our three examples of black men with substance dependencies. But often 'doing good' can come into conflict with autonomy—especially when an elder has no one with whom to consult about his or her best interests. You may want to grant an elder information in order to make a decision, though if that patient believes just talking about an adverse outcome will make it happen, autonomy may not be beneficent.

"First, do no harm," the medical rule, is more relevant here. But even avoidance of harm can be misinterpreted by some traditional AA elders if they are not given explanations. For example, a closed-chest compression may be viewed by a patient as malevolent if it is misunderstood.

Should patients and clients be told everything? What about ethnic elders? Some Ethiopian immigrants, for instance, believe that bad medical news should be conveyed by a family member or a close friend, not a health-care provider. A family insisting on silence can inhibit legal disclosure; a family insisting that a family member be present may inhibit confidentiality.

When someone does not wish to know a diagnosis or details, the information can be "titrated" (given only as requested). But a recent study found that patients of lower socioeconomic status asked fewer questions, thus giving providers the impression that they had little desire for information (Waitzkin, 1984), and this caused some clinicians to feel ethically justified in benevolently withholding bad news.

Fidelity

Close to beneficent honesty and autonomy is fidelity that embraces confidentiality. It remains imperative, but it has becoming increasingly difficult in an age of networking specialties, insurance verifications, and legal requirements. Also, confidentiality may be overridden if there is a risk of suicide, homicide, or danger to the general good, or (in certain cases) if it involves sexually transmitted diseases.

Faithfulness to the relationship can also entail giving attention to justice, including decisions about the rightful allocation of health and social resources. Today, in the United States, allocation is supposedly based on an assumption of the equality of each patient and on distribution according to need.

Relationship Skills

Blacks and whites may bring different expectations to counseling; most bear on outcome. Often, blacks evaluate the counseling relationship in terms of interpersonal skills (attentiveness to moods and responses; the dynamics, or flow, of events; and language) instead of instrumental skills (a focus on the results of an event or task, and achievement of a goal.) Gibbs's model (1981) of a constructive interpersonal counseling relationship with a black client included five stages.

In *stage one,* appraisal, the client sizes up the counselor and minimizes the intensity of the interaction. Do not confuse this with aloofness, hostility, or inability to verbalize. Distancing provides space to evaluate the counselor in terms of honesty and genuineness. It took Otis Brown a long time to trust his caseworker.

Two frustrated case managers had preceded Rose Dickson, his current worker; they had tried to help Mr. Brown see how unhealthy his lifestyle was and to offer help, but he had "kicked them out." They had told him his place was a mess and he needed homemaker help, that he was malnourished and needed meals on wheels, that he needed someone to help him bathe and take his medicine. They were right, but he had just waved his cane at them.

Rose Dickson tried a different tack. She too was black, and she had been raised in a large family that had its share of prideful, authoritarian men. She deferred to Mr. Brown's wishes. On her first visit, after some informal, neutral conversation about his past life, she shared some information about her own relatives, who had come up from the south. They both laughed about how hard it was to get used to the cold. Ms. Dickson ignored the squalor of Mr. Brown's home but asked if he was hungry. Would he mind if she brought in something from McDonalds? Later, fed and in a better mood, he listened while she told him about her agency's services—if he desired any of them. Laughing, she said she couldn't bring food from McDonalds every day, but there was a meals program he might consider. And there was some homemaker help. She didn't press the matter. She simply left her appointment card with a phone number, in case he needed to contact her sooner.

In the ensuing months, Ms. Dickson visited Mr. Brown weekly—always by appointment. She learned that he loved licorice and often would bring him some as a surprise. He looked forward to her visits and seemed perkier now that he was eating better. He hadn't realized that the meals program had soul food now and then. He also came to accept a personal care worker, and he was bathing regularly. "Next," he complained, "they'll be cleaning up this place and it won't even feel like home anymore." Ms. Dickson laughed—it was up to him, but both knew he would come around. He told her about his days in the army and the travel experiences the army had given him. "Here comes my listening girl," he would say when she arrived, "I hope you don't get sick of my stories." Sometimes he talked about his daughter, Marcella.

As Mr. Brown's basic needs were being met, Ms. Dickson's long-term goal was to encourage a medical checkup and then try to contact Marcella. She spent much time listening to him talk about "nonsense doctors not being worth a damn." She remained neutral but empathic. When she asked if she could arrange a doctor's appointment, he refused. She teased him, saying that he was a stubborn man but, again, that it was his decision. One night, Ms. Dickson received a call from his friend Betty Smith, who said that she had stopped by and found Mr. Brown on the floor. A rescue squad took him to an ER; his hip was broken. Ms. Dickson rushed over to the hospital. She knew that a new treatment plan would have to be devised for him now.

When you encounter resistance to your services, Jackson's (1983) advice is not to take this at face value but to view it as a reflexive defense in a struggle for identity or in a threateningly racist situation. With each other, blacks are open, responsive, playful, and expressive. Therefore, a goal of treatment may be to help the client find more self-serving adaptive strategies.

In *stage two,* there is a search for egalitarianism. A black client may become more assertive, asking personal questions—say, about beliefs—to decide if the counselor is able to go beyond stereotypes, power, and dominance. This is the appropriate time to deal with issues of race (Gibbs, 1981; Jones & Seagull, 1981).

You can model openness by examining your own feelings first; pretending will only make a problematic situation worse. "The ethnic competence model," wrote Green (1995), "calls for veracity, a simple and straightforward statement that race, ethnicity, or general background may be an issue and it should be clarified" (p. 201).

In *stage three,* the client may try to advance the relationship by asking for favors, mutual obligations, or exchanges of information, or by identifying with the worker personally rather than professionally. This can be difficult for professionally trained workers who have been taught otherwise.

In *stage four,* the client commits to a plan of service. The client's language may still be personal—for instance, expressing personal regard for you—and may indicate a willingness to consider your recommendations.

In *stage five,* Gibbs wrote, the engaged client moves from appraising you interpersonally to appraising your instrumental competence. This may be in conflict with your agency's modus operandi (a need to gather data; short-term, highly focused interventions); and to achieve ethnic competence, you may have to juggle interpersonal and instrumental styles.

Throughout, the gerocounselor will keep in mind the cultural contrasts between many families in the AA and Anglo American communities, for the client functions in both. For example, in the Anglo community, elders usually try to maintain independence from adult children and do not wish to be "a burden." In AA communities, the interdependent, fluid family is typically expected to take in or move in with an older person in order to continue an ongoing reciprocal arrangement. When these expectations are unmet, despair and intergenerational stress can result (Green, 1995).

How black patients relate to their physicians may provide some clues about their relationships with counselors. Mouton and associates (1995) identified four common models of the relationship between a physician and an AA patient: paternalistic, informative, deliberative, and interpretive.

In the *paternalistic model,* the physician is the patient's medical guardian. This model is often adopted by AA elders sharing autonomy with a perceived authority figure. In the *informative model,* the physician is a reporter and executor of technical information. This model tends to limit the caring approach that many AAs prefer. In the *deliberative model,* the physician helps the patient choose the best intervention, in terms of values. This model runs a risk of moral coercion or paternalism. These authors endorsed the *interpretive model,* in which an intervention is selected after the clinician, acting as adviser, helps the patient express his or her values: "Judging African Americans by a culturally sensitive model will increase the chance for proper interpretation and good decision making" (p. 116).

Countertransference

Countertransference—a result of positive and negative experiences with elders and minorities as well as naiveté, ignorance, or racism—can cause a counselor to act paternal, awkward, blundering, or even destructive. The counselor may try to use street slang, may become self-effacing, or may act apologetic for being white and privileged. Another may propose a "we versus they" stance that is also unhelpful. Counselors who are uncomfortable may engage in name-dropping about black sports or entertainment figures—a variation on an old theme: "Some of my best friends are . . ." These approaches are soon recognized as phony (Davis, 1984).

Although your own family customs may be deemed by the dominant society as "most effective," you should not necessarily impose them on others as *the way* a functional family should behave. For example, the members of a white nuclear family usually eat together; in black extended families, that may not happen so often, because adults work or are away—elders or children often take meals with other relatives or alone.

But white counselors do not have to abandon all of their usual effective interpersonal skills in a heroic or theatrical effort to earn the trust of a black clients. If you are not black, your job will be to acknowledge your different ethnic background early on. Ask if it causes the client discomfort. When you do this, you will be learning about the client's cultural rules, ways, and differences.

Hines and Boyd-Franklin (1982) warned about burnout. Inner-city families, white or black, with multiple problems can be so complex as to induce burnout. In counseling such families, try a team approach. Use a double mirror and consult the team after explaining to the family what you are doing, how, and why. Remember that in systems work, you do not have to solve all of the problems. Unless you are in a public service agency where you must schedule regular appointments, you may be limited to just a few sessions. However, a simple change in one area will create changes in other areas, so be grateful for even minor progress; you are not going to turn around several generations of family problems in one gallant effort.

Transference

Many poor blacks, like Otis, will be ambivalent about counseling services, having experienced years of snooping social workers who control benefits, police and judicial personnel who exert imperfect justice, and peers who associated counseling with craziness. You can explore this transference by asking about past experiences with counseling-type contacts, and you may be able to orient your geroclients to mental health practices and to dispel myths that may discourage them from becoming engaged. This means that you will have to extend yourself, meet them on their own turf, reassure them that you are not there to blame or judge, and show respect (do not use first names without permission).

However, the idea that all blacks have a negative view of counseling is a myth. Various studies show that AAs in general believe that help can be obtained, that both black and white counselors can be helpful, that counseling is more than just talking, and that a goal of counseling is self-understanding. Both black males and (slightly more) females have expressed comfort with counseling. It is the process itself that may cause problems. Sue and Sue (1990) wrote that 50 percent of black patients terminated therapy after the first session (compared with 30 percent of whites) for the following reasons:

(1) The counselor's racism, prejudice, superior attitude, or igno-rance may cause the counselor to limit treatment options, to focus only on intra-psychic conflicts, not, examine external influences, to fail to acknowledge positive strengths, or to take a blame-the-victim approach.

(2) The counselor's color blindness may cause the counselor to ignore differences, not explore race and culture, and come up with unrealistic middle-class strategies.

(3) The counselor's paternalism may cause the counselor to see every problem as a race or minority issue, thus excusing severe disorders or behaviors, not examining the client's contributions to the problem, fostering dependency, and preventing effective prob-lem-solving.

(4) The counselor's unquestioning acceptance of black power that says—because of racism, the client has the right to be hostile and act without considering the rights and feelings of others—may reinforce the client's dysfunctional behavior. Often this defense is an attempt to disprove racial guilt. (p. 219)

Communication Skills

Another myth is that AA families are nonverbal. They are very expressive—even verbose—among themselves in their own milieu. If inexpressiveness is seen, as many counselors attest, it could be a form of "cultural paranoia," a learned survival mechanism to be used with a distrusted white society. If, in counseling, you find that family communication is vague and confusing, try working with smaller subgroups and watch for nonverbal cues.

Ethnogerocounseling Assessment

A dual perspective—from both black and white culture—is neces-sary for understanding black elders and their families. Without such a perspective, there is a risk that AA clients will be errone-ously labeled "defective" in some way. Begin by remembering that the AA category is not homogeneous; you must discover intra-group differences and assess strengths as well as deficits. Marie's children, for instance, wanted her to have counseling, to Marie this meant another shameful experience.

In working with poor inner-city blacks, you will want to make an ecological assessment of transactions between individuals and of systems within and outside their neighborhoods. How does an existing support system, such as a black church, offer senior citizens services—for example, day programs, credit unions, and training in survival? Assessment should also include the availability of resources such as food and housing, family strengths, and community facilities and how they can be better utilized. Are external systems (welfare, courts, schools, Medicaid and Medicare, food stamps, and public housing) coordinated?

Here, you will guide your clients to available resources, and survival will take precedence over individual and family conflicts. If you are working with a family, your emphasis may be on how that family can most effectively coordinate and work with all of the necessary services.

As you get to know your clients, you may have to reassess your own preconceptions of black families if you have expected them to be deficient, with many problems. You will find that many are flexible, effective groups dealing well with racism, unemployment, and poverty. Perhaps they show more complexity than pathology. Some family characteristics that you will probably assess are:

1. Frequency of family aid.
2. Relationships between haves and have-nots.
3. Male-female relationships.
4. Values imparted to children.
5. Spiritual resources and how these are utilized.
6. Race consciousness: a source of pride, inspiration, and commitment to social change? (Martin & Martin, 1985).

You will no doubt be asking many questions in order to determine eligibility; but understand that uneducated inner-city blacks may become suspicious, having learned to distrust the government workers who checked up on them in the past. Like Rose Dickson, handle questions sensitively and do not assess distrust as psychopathology.

As already stated, misdiagnosis and mistreatment are common among minorities; and because AAs are often erroneously thought to be nonverbal, many have been denied "talking" therapy, although many can benefit from it if it is culturally sensitive and problem-oriented. Ben Wells's adult children firmly believe that

Ben would be alive today if he had been properly diagnosed and given counseling.

Physical Assessments

Nurses should learn to recognize color-related changes in dark-skinned patients. Bloch (1981) devised a color change assessment guide for determining certain medical problems unique to black patients.

Psychological Assessment

Azibo (1989), frustrated by what he considered a Eurocentric model of normality in *DSM IV* and *ICD* (International Classification of Diseases) constructed his own Afrocentric Azibo Nosology, listing 18 distinct disorders unique to the AA personality. He considered "normal" the black person who: (1) recognized himself or herself as African, (2) prioritized African interests and development, (3) respected and perpetuated all things African, and (4) supported conduct that neutralized anything anti-African. A black psychiatric disorder, Azibo believed, is a psychological misorientation or non-Afrocentric state—genetic blackness without psychological blackness (p. 305).

Sue and Sue (1990) suggested a number of assessment goals for black clients:

* Identify expectations about counseling, you, and the agency.
* Define confidentiality between you and referral source.
* Explore clients' feelings about your racial differences.
* Assess and discuss clients' modes of self-disclosure.
* Learn the history of a problem and the client's perception of it.
* Elicit information about family support.
* Identify strengths of the client and family in handling past problems.
* Explore external contributing problems (related to race, health, education, employment) and resources (agencies, religious organizations).
* Explore issues and conflicts involving racial identity.
* Establish mutually agreed-upon goals.

- Agree on the number of sessions and responsibilities of each party.
- Solicit the client's opinion about your ability to work together; if it is negative, consider other options.
- Be open, honest, authentic, and empathic, and use an individual approach for each person. (p. 225)

Ethnogerocounseling Goals

The process, goals, and expectations of white middle-class counselors (who constitute the majority of counselors today) may have to be altered to meet the worldviews, expectations, and ways of elder minority clients. The focus may of necessity be on external conditions such as housing, food stamps, or medical care rather than in-depth counseling. Solomon (1976) wrote that because black powerlessness is a more virulent stressor than individual dynamics, empowerment should be a more important goal of treatment than reducing anxiety.

Choosing Ethnogerocounseling Modalities

Family Counseling

Counseling is effective with black families when it is based on an extended family system, not a nuclear family system, even though family therapy with low-income blacks has, on the average, not been successful. In one study, the dropout rate for blacks was 81 percent, compared with 50 percent for white middle-class families. The main reasons given were fear that family secrets would be revealed and fear of criticism from the counselor. Boyd (1982) suggested that the counselor work with the original family structure and make it more functional rather than try to change it. Sacred principles of family therapy, such as attention to role assignments, boundaries, and hierarchies, will differ, so don't discount families that do not fit into traditional forms. True, role flexibility can cause problems if roles conflict or are obscure; but everybody may be parenting children and elderly family members may be the responsibility of collective efforts. Don't fall into the

trap of labeling such differences pathological. Flexible patterns
have been responsible for many families' very survival, and for
their strengths.

In assembling participants for family counseling, include all significant others, particularly males not in residence. Many are in
and out of the home or live away but are in close intimate contact.
A black woman client with whom I worked often referred to a
godson, a grandnephew (both in other states), and a separated
husband who were all viable members of her extended family and
had much influence over her decisions and well-being.

In setting up sessions, remember that many clients will not be able
to take time off from work, so you may have to make appointments
at odd times or use phone or letter contacts creatively. Some clients
may be leery about coming because they fear contact with a bureau-
cracy; some may view a home visit as "being checked up on" while
others may see it as a friendly outreach. Get advice from your elder
client or key family members and, if possible, be flexible.

Some family members may think you are asking them to come
because you blame them for the problem. Explain that you don't,
but that you do believe they are important in the elder's support
system and their input is valuable. They know the person better
than others, and the problem will ultimately be affecting them too.
Owing to distrust and inconvenience, you may not be able to get
all of the key members in, so do not be insistent. Visit them in
their own surroundings, and work with those you can get.

Don't expect to gather data in the first session; it will be enough
to establish rapport and get some family consensus about the
problem. A genogram (Burlingame, 1995) is an informal way of
gathering family data. It will probably be quite complex and not
along bloodlines. To uncover important support persons, ask, "Who
can you depend on for help when needed?" Still, be aware that a
family may be reluctant to share facts that reveal secrets such as
illegitimate births, cohabitation, incarcerations, and paternity. Enid
Maxwell never shared information about Daniel's father, and her
counselors did not ask.

Group Counseling

Group counseling can be just as effective with black elders and
their families as any other category. AAs are coping with the same

problems as all late-life families and benefit from information, stress management, and support when such aids reflect black values. Marie's religious values—not her black values—made it difficult for her to share in her alcoholic recovery groups; she could not get beyond the issue of shame. Through the years, I had several black older women in my racially mixed but mostly white middle-class senior support groups, and the AA women not only fit in well and benefited but also made excellent contributions as role models.

The Ecological Perspective

This perspective, which treats environmental as well as emotional problems, is generally most effective for low-income families. Counselors should cooperate with nonprofessionals and indigenous helpers, make frequent home visits, help clients access services, and carefully plan brief, short-term family tasks (Gwyn & Kilpatrick, 1981).

Ethnogerocounseling Interventions

Black social workers are often critical of the dominant culture's social work emphasis on intrapsychic states and talking therapy instead of making changes in the social and physical environment and dealing with its stressors (Devore & Schlesinger, 1991).

Jackson (1983) wrote that problems with multiple origins require multiple approaches. This widens the responsibilities of several black primary units: client and family; professional counselor; community, cultural, political, and economic systems; and the general environment, with special emphasis on the family and racial group.

The aim of any intervention is to help the black client understand the problem and facilitate behaviors that are compatible with black culture. As mentioned, assessment should include the clients' opinions about the provider's credibility, competence, and motivation—for even a counselor who is black may be seen as an extension of the white system, influenced by racism.

Interventions for personal growth or changes in behavior, perception, cognition, or the environment should be done according to your assessment of the elder's personal and cultural values.

Thus race, black identity, and black culture are cornerstones of Jackson's model. Barriers may include a lack of creative funding and support networks, the professional's fear of taking risks and abandoning economic advantages, and the vast variability of black people.

Berlin and Fowkes (1983) developed a cross-cultural model for services to minorities using the acronym LEARN:

Listen to patient's perception of problem.

Explain your professional perception of problem.

Acknowledge, discuss differences and similarities.

Recommend intervention or treatment.

Negotiate agreement. (p. 935)

These authors wrote that most black families responded well to time-limited, problem-solving, family systems approaches in which the counselor was active, direct, and goal-oriented. Insight into causes may be unnecessary; results are needed. Concentrate on the conditions that are maintaining the problem in order to change them; and focus on what family members say and how they react to one another and to your interventions.

If a black family is involved in a religious organization, enlist a clergyman or -woman to help with family issues (with the client's permission). Also, consider the role of religious organizations and other organizations in the community. For instance, can church enrichment programs be developed for families or elders? Can adult education classes be started to discuss elder care and form support groups? Advertise to get extended families to attend, because they are probably involved too. Recruit skilled black adults who have weathered similar storms to discuss their experiences and help other families. Include home visits for more effective communication.

As discussed, since the lot of black men is sometimes different from that of black women, you may wish to offer different treatment options for them. Some men, black or other, are often unprepared or unwilling to share personal problems with strangers—especially with whites—and they are often resistant to counseling, considering it a threat or a sign of weakness. June (1986) recommended that counselors and agency personnel be trained in culturally sensitive communication and counseling skills by black professionals as part of an aggressive outreach effort to reach more AA men.

Reminiscence and life review can be effective ways to help ethnic elders examine their personal histories and create a sense of accomplishment and predictability. Otis Brown told Rose about a lifetime of struggle but also about rewarding, positive experiences that helped him generate a sense of integrity about his life. This may not be as easy for a counselor who, unlike Rose, does not know of the traditions of the AA community or who is much younger. In getting started, it may help to share with clients the Historical Context at the beginning of this part, and to discuss their impressions of those events, adding your own perceptions. This will be not only a life review but also "validation therapy"; as you validate a life that moved through important times. "There is a need for more than a sympathetic ear or polite reinforcement; active listening based on cultural knowledge and skills in ethnographic interviewing is needed" (Green, 1995, p. 204).

Ethnogerocounseling Terminations

As with all older clients, work with AA elders will include terminating interviews, cases, and counseling relationships as some clients move to different levels of care and some die.

End-of-life issues are perceived and handled differently by various cultures. Some AA elders, for example, refuse care after receiving a diagnosis of a terminal illness; but—more than whites—they have been found to disapprove of allowing people who want to die do so, or to stop life-prolonging treatments (Caralis, 1993).

A chaplain to suffering and dying black elders, Rev. Malvina Stephens (1995), described herself as spiritual caregiver in an almost mystical or spiritual relationship with the sick person. The touch of a caregiver's hand, she said, "is like a touch of God giving strength." The spiritual caregiver becomes a mediator to God, appealing on the patient's behalf. It is common for religious people to feel angry with God and to ask, "Why me? Why now? How will I be remembered? What do I leave posterity? Why did God let this happen to me? What is life worth?" The spiritual caregiver has no pat answers but helps the person to explore and resolve some common spiritual problems, such as a loss of meaning in life, loss of a former belief system, and anger with God. Sometimes the spiritual caregiver just sits silently with the family through the journey to death.

AARP (1990a) warns that you must take a practical as well as religious or psychological approach when a widowed person is withdrawing and isolated. This may not be a manifestation of culture or bereavement; rather, isolation is often caused by financial problems due to the death of a spouse. When money is curtailed in an already straitened situation, isolation and loneliness will be magnified, and the person may need concrete as well as psychological assistance (p. 6).

EXERCISE
Think again about the black elders who are described at the beginning of this chapter part. On the basis of some of the principles of ethnogerocounseling discussed here, how would you devise a care or treatment plan for each person? How would you proceed? What would you include? What more do you need to know? Include both micro and macro interventions.

References for Part IV

American Association of Retired Persons. (1990a). *Customs of bereavement: A guide for providing cross-cultural assistance.* Washington, DC: AARP.

American Association of Retired Persons. (1990b). *Health risks and preventive care among older blacks.* Washington, DC: AARP.

American Association of Retired Persons Minority Affairs (1995). *A Portrait of older minorities.* Washington, DC: AARP.

Azibo, D. (1989). African-centered themes on mental health and nosology of Black/African personality disorder. *Journal of Black Psychology, 15* (2), 173–214.

Baker, F. (1991). Background on mental health and mental illness from the perspective of the African American elder. In Working Paper, Palo Alto, CA: Stanford Geriatric Education Center.

Baldwin, J. (1984). African self-consciousness and the mental health of African Americans. *Journal of Black Studies, 15* (2), 177–194.

Barnes, E. (1972). The black community as the science of positive self concept for black children: A theoretical perspective. In R. Jones (Ed.), *Black psychology.* New York: Harper and Row.

Berlin, E., & Fowkes, W. (1983). A teaching framework for cross-cultural health care. *Western Journal of Medicine, 139* (6), 934–938.

Bloch, B. (1981). Nursing care of black patients. In M. S. Orque, B. Bloch, & L. Monrroy (Eds.), *Ethnic nursing care: A multicultural approach,* pp. 81–113. St. Louis, MO: Mosby.

Boyd, N. (1982). Family therapy with black families. In E. Jones & S. Korchin (Eds.), *Minority mental health.* New York: Praeger, pp. 227–249.

Burlingame, V. (1995). *Gerocounseling: Counseling elders and their families.* New York: Springer.

Caralis, P. (1993). The influence of ethnicity and race on attitudes toward advance directives. *Journal of Clinical Ethics, 4,* 155–165.

Daly, J., Jennings, J., Beckett, J. & Leashore, B. (1995). Effective coping strategies of African Americans. *Social Work Journal of the National Association of Social Workers, 40* (2), 240–248.

Davis, L. (1984). *Ethnicity in social work practice.* New York: Haworth.

Delany, S. & Delany, E. (1993). *Having our say.* New York: Kodansha International.

Devore, W., & Schlesinger, E. (1991). *Ethnic-sensitive social work practice* (3rd ed.). New York: Merrill (Macmillan).

Du Bois, W. (1903). *The souls of black folk.* New York: Author. Reprinted 1961, Fawcett Publications, Inc.

Edmonds, M. M. (1994). Black women today. Presentation at Stanford Medical School, Palo Alto, CA (video tape).

Erickson, E. (1950). *Childhood and society.* New York: Norton.

Gibbs, J. (1981). The interpersonal orientation in mental health consultation: toward a model of ethnic variations in consultation. In R. Dana (Ed.), *Human services for cultural minorities.* Baltimore, MD: University Park Press.

Green, J. (1995). *Cultural awareness in the human services: A multi-ethnic approach.* Boston: Allyn and Bacon.

Gwyn, F., & Kilpatrick, A. (1981). Family therapy with low-income blacks: A tool or a turn-off? *Social Casework 62,* 259–266.

Hale-Benson, J. (1982). *Black children: Their roots, culture, and learning styles.* Baltimore, MD: Johns Hopkins University Press.

Haley, A. (1976). *Roots*. Garden City, NY: Doubleday.

Hines, P. & Boyd-Franklin, N. (1982). Black families. In M. McGoldrick, J. Pearce, & J. Giordano (Eds.), *Ethnicity and family therapy*. New York: Guilford, pp. 84–107.

Hooyman, N., & Kiyak, H. (1996). *Social gerontology: A multidisciplinary perspective* (3rd ed.). Boston: Allyn and Bacon.

Jackson, A. (1983). A theoretical model for the practice of psychotherapy with Black populations. *Journal of Black Psychology, 10,* 19–27.

Jackson, J. J. (1975). Plight of older women in the United States. *Black Aging, 1,* 12–20.

Jackson, J. S. (1991). *Life in black America*. Newbury Park, CA: Sage.

Jones, A., & Seagull, A. (1981). Dimensions of the relationship between the black client and the white therapist: A theoretical overview. *American Psychologist, 32,* 850–855.

June, L. (1986). Enhancing the delivery of mental health and counseling services to black males: Critical agency and provider responsibilities. *Journal of Multicultural Counseling and Development, 14,* 39–44.

Locke, D. (1992). *Increasing multicultural understanding*. Newbury Park, CA: Sage.

Martin, J., & Martin, E. (1985). *The helping tradition in the black family and community*. Silver Spring, MD: National Association of Social Workers.

Medearis, A. (1994). *The African American kitchen*. NY: Dutton/Penguin.

Meyers, H., & King, L. (1983). Mental health issues in the development of the black American child. In G. Powell (Ed.), *The psychosocial development of minority group children*. New York: Brunner/Mazel, pp. 275–306.

Mouton, C., Johnson, M., & Cole, D. (1995). Ethical considerations with African-American elders. *Clinics in Geriatric Medicine, 11* (1), 113–129.

National Caucus and Center on Black Aged. (1984). *The status of the black elderly in the United States*. A report for the Select Committee on Aging, House of Representatives. Committee Publication No. 100–622.

Norton, D. (1983). Black family life patterns, the development of self and cognitive development of black children. In G. Powell (Ed.), *The psychosocial development of minority group children*. New York: Brunner/Mazel, pp. 181–193.

Powell, G. (1983). Coping with adversity: The psychosocial development of Afro-American children. In G. Powell (Ed.), *The psychosocial development of minority group children*. New York: Brunner/Mazel, pp. 49–76.

Richardson, J. (1990). *Aging and health: Black American elders*. SGEC Working Papers Series, No. 4. Palo Alto, CA: Stanford Geriatric Education Center.

Solomon, B. (1976). *Black empowerment: Social work in oppressed communities*. New York: Columbia University Press.

Stephens, M. (1995). Spiritual concerns of the dying. Panel discussion presentation at the Cultural Diversity and End of Life Issues Conference, Stanford, CA: Stanford Geriatric Education Center.

Sue, D., & Sue, S. (1990). *Counseling the culturally different* (2nd ed.). New York: Wiley.

Taylor, R., & Chatters, L. (1991). Religious life. In J. Jackson (Ed.), *Life in black America*. Newbury Park, CA: Sage.

Valentine, C. (1971). Deficit, differences and bicultural models of Afro-American behavior. *Harvard Educational Review, 41*, 137–157.

Waitzkin, H. (1984). Doctor-patient communication. *Journal of the American Medical Association, 252*–261.

Wilson, W. (1987a). *The developmental psychology of the black child*. New York: Africana Research Publications.

Wilson, W. (1987b). *The truly disadvantaged: The inner city, the underclass, and public policy*. Chicago: University of Chicago Press.

Yeo, G., & Gallagher-Thompson, D. (1996). *Ethnicity and the dementias*. Bristol, PA: Taylor and Francis.

Young, R., Kahana, E., & Waller, J. (1988). *Racial aspects of caregiving strain over time*. Paper presented at the 41st Annual Scientific Meeting of the Gerontology Society of America, San Francisco, CA.

Acknowledgments for Part IV

I thank the Geriatric Education Centers at Stanford University (SGEC), Palo Alto, California, and at Marquette University (WGEC), Milwaukee, Wisconsin, for generously sharing hard-to-get current literature on ethnicity, aging, and African-American families. Many individuals also helped in the preparation of this chapter. I wish to also thank the gracious AA health and social service providers and others who took time out of their busy schedules to grant me interviews or presented material at workshops that I attended.

From California: Elwood Jackson, Director of the Bell Park Community Center in East Palo Alto; Maud August, Director of the Temple Arms Center in Oakland; Julee Richardson, PhD, Coordinator, Older Adult Education Program at Chabot College in Hayward and faculty, SGEC; and E. Percil Stanford, PhD, San Diego State University. From New York City: Elizabeth Geary, MSW, Program Director; and Sandra Christian, MSW, at Lenox Hill Neighborhood House. From Florida: Bob Bozonne, MA, Executive Director; and Cathy Claud, Director, CARP Domiciliary Program in Fort Worth, and staff members at Hanley-Hazelden at St. Mary's in West Palm Beach.

People in Wisconsin who helped: Romana Dicks-Williams, MSW, Case Manager, Milwaukee Department of Aging; Corrine Owens, MA, retired teacher and civil rights activist, Rev. Norma Carter, Pastor, Gospel Assembly Church of Racine; Joan Dyess, member, Racine County Minority Task Force on Aging; and Lorena Harris, retired teacher and NAACP volunteer.

PART V

Asian/Pacific Island (A/PI) Elders

Asians are . . .

        silent people

Never speaking of distress

Bearing much in their heart

The burden of the silent one.

Standing up to their rights

Trying to prove loyal by working hard.

America, a place of hopes

For white people only!

(Written by an Asian middle school student in 1973. From Powell, 1983, p. 164.)

Historical Context

1700	Small number of Filipinos immigrate to Louisana.
1701	Sojourner immigration by men from South China.
1870	Brutality; violence; discriminatory legislation.
1879	California constitution adopted, with anti-Chinese provisions.
1882	Chinese Exclusion Act bans Chinese immigration. Immigration of "paper sons."
1890s	Japanese become second Asian group to immigrate.
1898	Spanish-American War ends; Philippine Islands are now a possession of the United States.
1900–1925	Rise of family associations and tongs.
1903	First wave of Filipino "Pensionados" immigrate. Filipinos recruited for Hawaiian plantations. Second wave of Filipinos to the west coast.
1914–1918	World War I.
1930	Great Depression.
1934	Tydings-McDuffie Act sets yearly quota of Filipinos at 50.
1939–1945	World War II. Over 110,000 Japanese Americans are interned with neither charges nor trials.
1940–1946	16,000 Chinese Americans serve in U.S. armed forces; Filipinos serve in U.S. army and navy.
1944	Japanese-American men drafted into segregated units.
1946	Philippines gain independence. American Filipinos and veterans are finally able to become citizens.
1947–1952	Over 9,000 Asian wives immigrate; high birthrates.
1953	Refugee status approved for 2,000 if approved by Taiwan.
1957–1975	Vietnam War; United States' intervention, 1964–1975.
1959	Hawaii becomes 50th state.
1965	Communist revolution in China creates distrust of A/PIs. Third wave of Filipino professionals immigrate. Older Americans Act passed.
1970s	American Chinese are divided between educated and uneducated. Immigration from Vietnam occurs.

1980s	"Model minority" image prevails.
	Heavy immigration from Hong Kong and Taiwan.
1983	United States admits grave injustice to Japanese-Americans.
1989	Tiananmen Square massacre.

Case Examples

Hulan Fu, a Middle-Class Chinese Woman With Medical Problems and Minimal Family Support

Hulan Fu, age 93, came to the United States in 1965 at age 61 to finally join her husband, Wen Fu, after a 50 year separation. Wen, a paper son who immigrated to the United States in 1900, married Hulan in China in 1920 but under the Chinese Exclusion Act of 1924, she was not allowed to join him here. Wen ran a laundry in Boston's West End and worked diligently for both money and immigration clearance. His wife's hoped-for passage came in 1965, when the ban was lifted.

Despite her years of waiting and preparation, the trip was stressful for Hulan—and her husband was a stranger. But she had looked forward to joining siblings and nieces and nephews in the new land (she herself was childless). She immediately embarked on English classes, joined a Chinese women's society, and baby-sat with family great grandchildren in the close-knit neighborhood. But often she felt overburdened by the baby-sitting and overwhelmed by language differences and other differences that now existed in her family. She felt that her life was out of balance. She also suffered severe backaches. She consulted Chinese doctors, who treated her pain with acupuncture and herbs. She improved somewhat but had recurring episodes of pain.

After her arrival, the Fus were evicted from their ethnic area to make way for new high-rise condos. Packing and relocating were hard for Hulan, and she injured her back again—this time so badly that she was taken to the ER at Massachusetts General Hospital. She was diagnosed with spinal fractures due to severe osteoporosis. Hulan combined Chinese medicine (yin) with American (yang) and improved. Wen's reaction to relocation was worse. He developed hypertension, had a stroke, and died two years later.

Hulan, now a widow, lives in a housing project in North Quincy. She is stooped and has developed heart disease. She has in-home health and social services, but family support is dwindling because family members have their own medical problems. She is increasingly isolated—an unusual situation in this ethnic population. A nursing home is being considered because she is often noncompliant about using American medicine paid by Medicare. However, Hulan says that a nursing home will kill her, and her relatives agree. They fear suicide.

Shon Young-Kim, Korean Male From A Poor Environment With Strong Family Support

Shon Young–Kim, 78, and wife, Hwaja, 75, immigrated to San Jose from Korea in 1975 to join their two sons. Hwaja, a shy, passive woman who never learned English, kept house; Shon, somewhat bilingual, worked as a gardener. At his retirement, he was eligible for SSI, MediCal, and HUD-subsidized senior housing.

Shon enjoyed American beer and increased his intake after his retirement. When drunk, he was mean and physically and verbally abusive to Hwaja. She never complained, nor did their Korean neighbors; but less timid neighbors called the police several times.

Whenever the domestic violence squad came, Hwaya and her Korean friends denied any abuse. They were embarrassed to be in trouble; it almost seemed they expected females to be abused. The police would scold Shon to drink less and treat Hwaya better, and then depart until the next time. On one call, they noticed Hwaya's bruises and jailed Shon. But denying any abuse, his sons bailed him out.

Mary V., the Senior Center Director, finally called in people from Adult Protective Services, who interviewed family members and encountered more denials. The case was dropped. The center's small Korean community handled the problem by shaming Shon for his drinking and avoiding him. They also apologized to their neighbors for his behavior. As Hwaja's screams continued, Ms. V. next contacted the Korean Senior Program, which sent a case manager to inform Shon that abuse was against the law. Shon did not allow Hwaja to speak with the worker. The denials continued.

Several months later, Shon was involved in a seemingly minor automobile accident, but Hwaja was thrown from the car and killed. Some people believe that Shon pushed her out, but this was never proved. The Senior Center Director felt frustrated and hopeless about this lost generation. She posted signs in Korean and other languages that read, "Elder abuse is against the law." But she decided that while strict intervention was necessary with these elders, the only real hope was in educating the next generation.

Tony Mulos, a Middle-Class Filipino With Depression and Minimal Family Support

Tony Mulos is age 76. At age 29, as a veteran, he qualified to immigrate to the United States from the northern Phillipines. A high school graduate, he spoke both English and Ilocano. Mr. Mulos found work in the service industry, married, divorced, and then settled south of Market Street in San Francisco—alone, until he remarried in 1965. He and his second wife, Dolores, were childless. She died of cancer when he was 70. He had lovingly nursed her through her illness, but the stress aggravated his hypertension and his tendency to isolate himself.

Neighbors expected Mr. Mulos to be depressed when his wife died; but when he did not improve after 2 years, they were concerned. He had become emaciated and lifeless-looking. One neighbor discussed her concerns with her own case manager, and Peter F. from the Philippine Outreach Program of the Department of Mental Health was called in.

Peter F. was sensitive to Mr. Mulos's pride and to his other ethnic customs. He did not speak in terms of mental illness but simply said that such a shy, quiet, and now sad man perhaps needed some medicine to give him more energy to do things. (The word "depression" was never used.) Mr. Mulos agreed, for the sake of increasing his energy.

Once Mr. Mulos was on an antidepressant medication, Peter F. called weekly, speaking in the Ilocano dialect. Mr. Mulos imagined that these were just friendly calls, but actually they were a form of therapy. He told the counselor about his homeland, the army, his hardships in the United States, and now his loneliness. The counselor supported him and suggested that he attend the Philippine Senior Center to play cards and bingo, and to dance. Mr. Mulos refused initially, but with continued prompting, he agreed to go once with the counselor.

Mr. Mulos enjoyed the center, where he soon met Rose A., who also spoke the Ilocano dialect. She was a pleasant widow with five daughters and sixteen grandchildren. They eventually married, and now Mr. Mulos is the patriarch of a large family, like the one he had always dreamed about (even though his wife indirectly runs the show).

Mee Lee, a Hmong Woman From a Poor Environment With Dementia and Strong Family Support

Mee Lee is an 82-year-old Hmong Laotian woman. Along with 10 other family members, she joined her husband's large clan in southeast Wisconsin in 1980, after spending 2 difficult years in a refugee camp in Thailand. Her immigration was sponsored by a cousin and Lutheran Social Services in Wisconsin. Because of language and age problems, neither she nor her husband became formally employed (or became citizens). They were supported by the family-clan, Medicaid, and SSI. They lived with their oldest son at first. Later, when HUD housing was available, they moved nearby. They continued to receive daily support and communication from the family. They joined a Hmong group at a senior center and enjoyed the center's bingo and trips.

In 1994, Mrs. Lee became increasingly forgetful and combative. Her family attributed this to her age and her very strong personality. Unusual for a Hmong woman, she was headstrong all her life. In 1996, her husband, Yong, died of heart disease. The family (mostly her daughter-in-law, Kia) then assumed more caregiving responsibilities. Mrs. Lee moved in with her son. Her dementia has since progressed. Now, it is hard for her family to care for her, as she wanders and must be watched constantly. Her agitation and combativeness are worse and her relatives—who understand little of her diagnosis, Alzheimer's disease—feel that she is being difficult on purpose.

Mrs. Lee sometimes strikes her daughter-in-law, who is overworked, overwhelmed, and sad but nonetheless cares for her faithfully. The case manager, Mary O'Brien, has suggested formal day treatment, respite care, or even a nursing home, but the family refuses even to consider such options. She has also tried to explain Alzheimer's disease but does not believe she is getting through to them. Ms. O'Brien sees Kia Lee going downhill; knowing the odds, she fears that she will soon be dealing with two sick people if the family does not accept help. She is frustrated and doesn't know where to turn.

Now new problems have arisen. Benefit cuts are being threatened for noncitizen immigrants. Mrs. Lee's son was injured in an accident last year and lost many work days. The family is in debt. Mrs. Lee's maintenance will be an added burden to this already stressed family.

Chapter 13

The A/PI Ethnic Lens

Asian and Pacific Island American (A/PI), a political term designed for a strength-in-numbers effect, was coined in the 1960s to unite the divergent American nationality groups of Asia and the Pacific Islands into a United States census category. The term *Oriental,* also political but coined by the British, is not preferred by most A/PIs today.

As you change to the A/PI Ethnic Lens, you will make corrections in your Gero Chi Model to accommodate the unique circumstances of these peoples: demographics, immigrations, relocations, cultural attributes, and special issues. But again a word of warning! We will be speaking of A/PIs as a broad category, and there are many intergroup and intragroup differences.

Identity

This widely heterogeneous category consists of over 20 distinct cultures, the largest being (in order) the Chinese, Filipinos, Japanese, Asian Indians, Indochinese (Vietnamese, Lao and Hmongs, Khmers), and Koreans. Among the Pacific Islanders (5 percent) are the Polynesians (Hawaiians, Samoans, Tongans), Micronesians (Chamorros from Guam, for example), and Melanesians (Figians, for example). We will focus primarily on the Chinese, Filipinos, Japanese, Indochinese, and Koreans. Asian Indians constitute the fourth-largest group, but there is little information on them at this time.

Demographics

The total numbers of A/PI elders grew 120 percent between the census of 1970 and the census of 1980, making them third-largest and the fastest-growing minority in the United States today. This rapid numerical increase is attributed to immigration, natural growth, and the fact that new racial definitions formulated since 1970 have caused more A/PIs to be counted (AARP, 1995).

Most A/PI elderly people, like Tony Bulos and the Kims, reside in California, followed by Washington, New York, Texas, Illinois, and New Jersey. Many Hmongs also live in Rhode Island, Minnesota, and Wisconsin, where Mee Lee now resides. Mr. and Mrs. Fu settled in Boston, Massachusetts.

A/PIs are commonly believed to be a "model minority" who work hard, who parallel white middle-class values, and who have therefore achieved the American dream of material and vocational success. True, the Chinese and Japanese especially exceed the national median income and educational status; but in 1990 that median income, ($7,906 for men and $6,570 for women 65 years and over) was only about half of the $14,775 income of white men in the same age group. (It was closer to the income for white women 65 and older, $8,297.) Of these A/PI elders, 13 percent live below the poverty level, compared with 10 percent whites; and fewer of those in poverty receive public assistance or welfare than people in other categories. The higher levels of income in the total A/PI population reflect households with two incomes, and some wages that are very high. About 16 percent over age 65 are employed (Sue & Sue, 1990).

While A/PIs appear to get into the best schools and earn the best grades, their educational profile includes a large uneducated mass with serious language problems and another large highly educated group often considered "underemployed" and "underpaid" relative to their education and training. Ten percent of older A/PIs have no formal education, compared with 1 percent of white elders.

Rates of intermarriage among members of the dominant society are higher for A/PIs than other minorities, signifying a decreasing social distance. Now, the majority of men 65 and over are married, and more A/PI women over 65 are married than their white counterparts.

There are few data on the health status of A/PIs, whose elders use fewer formal health services; but unrecognized cancers, hypertension, and tuberculosis are high concerns. Statistics on mental health stats reveal them to be relatively well-adjusted and functioning effectively in American society, with few problems. Their overall rates of delinquency, crime, psychiatric admissions, and divorce are lower than those of any other category (Sue & Sue, 1990).

But these glowing statistics conceal some hard facts. While overall social problems appear statistically low, problems in ghetto areas—the Chinatowns, Koreatowns, and Japantowns of large American cities (where many elderly people live)—are enormous. The population density of San Francisco's Chinatown, for example, is second only to that of Harlem. Unemployment, poverty, health problems, juvenile delinquency, drugs, crime, and suicide run rampant in these overcrowded areas while mental health facilities continue to be underutilized (Sue & Sue, 1990).

Immigration and Migration Experiences

The circumstances and timing of one's immigration to the United States are often critical factors in successful adaptation, family harmony, and even one's future aging process. The Japanese, for example, have developed terms suggesting the importance of timing. A *Japanese national* is a person born in Japan, and an *issei* is a first-generation American, to some degree isolated from both American and Japanese culture. Second-generation Japanese—who in general were born between the two world wars—are called *nisei,* and their American-born children who were sent to Japan to be educated are called *kibei-nisei. Sansei* are postwar third-generation children educated here.

Chances are that your A/PI geroclients or their parents came to the United States in one of several waves of immigration.

ASIAN/PACIFIC ISLAND IMMIGRATIONS TO THE
UNITED STATES
1840s   Chinese Gold gold rush
1900s   Japanese, Filipino, etc.
Mid-1960s   Immigrants' families arrive
Mid-1970s   Indochinese immigrants and refugees
1990s   A/PI immigrations continue

The 1840s

The first significant number of Asian immigrants were single, poorly educated males from Kwangtung province in southern China, who came as cheap labor, filling a void created by the California gold rush and the building of the transcontinental railroad around 1840. Many had been led to believe they would make a fortune in the United States; some were sojourners who hoped to return home wealthy, and others planned to send for their families. But when their jobs ended, these Chinese workers were viewed as a threat to the diminished American labor market. An almost national mind-set resulted, based on white supremacy and Asian inferiority; it led to scapegoating of Asians and discrimination against them. They were harassed because of their "quaint" ways—their customs, pigtails, language, and diet—and also because of their adverse circumstances, such as crowded living quarters. Since jobs and money were scarce, Chinese railroad workers volunteered or were compelled to set the dynamite charges to clear rock. The saying "Not a Chinaman's chance" reflected this work, with its high risk of losing life or limb.

These strong feelings against the Chinese were the impetus for the Chinese Exclusion Act of 1882, which prohibited the entry, naturalization, and intermarriage of the Chinese at first, and then, in 1924, of all Asians. Most early Asian immigrants were single males, and this act—in conjunction with laws against miscegenation—prevented them from marrying and establishing families and created an impoverished bachelor society. Today, many of these now oldest men are still without family support.

The Wu family, from our examples, is illustrative. Wen Fu's father came to the United States in 1880 planning to work, get rich, and return to China for a bride. Coming on a credit ticket, he had borrowed $70 for his passage and expenses and owed the Hong Kong lenders $200—a sum he found impossible to save and repay once he was here. In 1882, under the Chinese Exclusion Act, even as a documented American citizen, Mr. Fu learned he was not allowed to bring a bride here but could return to China to marry and acquire a "paper son," and his own Wen Fu was born in 1885. Wen joined his father 15 years later, and the pair moved to Boston's West End, where they worked up a small laundry business. In 1915, Wen followed his father's footsteps and married Hulan in China, hoping for a "paper son" of his own to bring to the United States; but the marriage was childless. Wen visited Hulan several times and saved for her hoped-for passage, and she was finally able to join him legally in 1965, 50 years after their marriage.

The 1900s

Around 1890–1920, Japanese and Filipinos entered the United States in large numbers. Many of the Japanese had left their homeland because of economic hardships resulting from modernization, and they mainly found jobs in the railroads, canneries, mining, and agriculture. Segregated and not allowed to intermarry, they devised a system of matchmakers and arranged marriages involving exchanges of photos with Japanese 'picture brides.'

Many Filipino males worked on large Hawaiian plantations and in mainland businesses. Tony Bulos worked in the San Francisco service industry. But soon he, like others, met with discrimination from labor unions and other groups. For Filipinos too, the Immigration Act of 1924 created a lack of females and family caregivers and led to isolation and loneliness.

Some of the unemployed Chinese railroad workers moved to jobs in fruit and vegetable markets, and many like Wen Fu, set up their own Chinese laundries. Today, many new immigrants open dry-cleaning and shoe repair businesses which require a minimum of English and in which the whole family can work together.

The Mid-1960s

Probably as a result of the civil rights movement and Americans' guilt about the ill-treatment of the Japanese Americans during

World War II, the Asian Immigration Acts of 1882 and 1924 were repealed in 1965. This allowed many Asian families and their aging relatives to be reunited. Many Koreans, like the Kims, immigrated here during this time; by 1985, there were over 542,000 Koreans working in small, family-centered businesses, mostly in Koreatown in Los Angeles.

The Mid-1970s

Since 1975, there has been an influx of immigrants and refugees from Indochina (southeast Asia). Having arrived in three separate waves, each with its own set of circumstances, they are ethnically very diverse. They include over 700,000 refugees, especially Vietnamese (66.6 percent), Khmers (20.5 percent), Laotians (13.5 percent), and Hmong (7.8 percent).

The first wave (1975) consisted of Vietnamese refugees who left abruptly after the fall of Saigon. Many of these southeast Asians were American government workers and businesspeople who were familiar with American culture, but they still arrived with high rates of depression.

In the second wave (1979–1982) were the "Boat people." They tended to be less educated, less-proficient in English, and less job skilled. They had endured severe trauma at home, in transit, and finally in various host countries; and they also experienced multiple losses and severe uncertainty regarding the whereabouts and safety of their kin. Mee Lee, for instance, spent 2 years in a refugee camp in Thailand before she was able to enter the United States with 10 members of her family.

The nurse Miva Yang and her family also came by boat, first to a settlement camp in Thailand, then to southern France, and later to Sheboygan, Wisconsin to join a settlement hosted by the Lutheran Church there. For them, the culture shock was enormous. At a presentation in Wausau, Yang showed slides of what it was like for most of the people like her: leaving a slow, primitive rural setting with dirt roads, and arriving suddenly in the fast-paced, urban sprawl of cities like Los Angeles—a step of 300 years virtually in an instant.

The third wave, consisting of mostly illiterate elders and unaccompanied minors, took place after the Orderly Departure Program in 1982. During the cold war, China's reputation in the

United States changed; Americans' attitude went from admiration to disenchantment (1944–1949) and then hostility (1949–1972). Nixon's visit to China in 1972 helped to soften this hostility; but the Tiananmen Square massacre in 1989 revived it.

The 1990s

Now, as A/PIs continue to immigrate to the United States, their numbers are expected to double by 2013—but some anti-immigration sentiment has reemerged, so this prediction may change. Filipinos are expected to become the largest group, followed by the Chinese, the Koreans, and then the Vietnamese (Sue & Sue, 1990).

Cultural Values

In the American media, A/PI culture has frequently been portrayed as quaint, sinister, or overly competitive and acquisitive. Here, it is again important to remind you that A/PIs, like all older persons, cannot be lumped together as a homogeneous group. There are over 20 different nationalities among them—there are over 29 distinct subgroups in the Chinese American population alone—and these peoples differ in language, religion, and customs. Also, Asian Americans born and bred in the United States who have assumed many of its cultural values differ from many elderly or newly immigrated A/PIs.

Still, there are some commonalities. Filial piety, smooth interpersonal relations, and reciprocity are observable and allow reasonable generalizations, not stereotypes, to be made. Accomplishments, correct behavior, and status are important measures of success; and the concept of flexible, important time is related to valuing personal and family events over other affairs (AARP, 1996).

The peoples of the Asian continent represent some of the world's oldest cultures and have had a profound influence on western art, architecture, and philosophy, despite the fact that several "closed door" political eras prevented cultural exchanges with the world. In this century, Asian American students and professionals are making landmark contributions in every field, particularly the sciences, mathematics, and electronics. The dedication of A/PIs in these fields has been attributed to the Asian work ethic and to innate talents, but it also is a successful accommodation to linguistic handicaps.

Many contrasts between eastern and western concepts are relevant to gerocounseling. One Asian model—which is gaining more attention in the United States—stresses daily spirituality rather than "weekend religion," balance and integration of mind and body rather than western dualism, a circular rather than a linear life orientation, preventive (yin) medicine rather than aggressive (yang) treatment, and reliance on self-help and indigenous remedies rather than synthetic drugs. As resources in the United States become scarcer and the medical needs of the elderly increase, it would not be surprising to see a continuing trend toward the eastern model. This can already be noted in the growing acceptance of alternative treatments such as tai chi, zen, meditation, deep breathing (chigon), acupuncture, and acupressure.

Asia has experienced recurrent droughts and famines, and perhaps because of this Asians eat a wide variety of foods and reject little. The Hans, China's largest ethnic group, have the most influence on the Chinese diet; but in Bejing, Muslim influences are also seen (the Muslims eat kid, horse, and donkey meat, but no pork). The main staple especially in the north is polished white rice. Few dairy products are consumed, but soy beans, called the "poor man's cow," are used to make soy sauce, milk, tofu, etc. Tea is popular; soda and coffee are gaining in popularity.

A balance of *fan* (grains served in a separate bowl for each dinner) and *ts'ai* (cooked vegetables and meats shared from bowls centered on the table) is usual. Meals served three times a day must have *fan* but can omit *ts'ai,* except at banquets and at very good restaurants, where the opposite is true. Much fish (called *sushi* when raw) is eaten in Japan; dog meat is common in Korea. Fruits are scarce everywhere.

In China, food is considered important to harmony and health, and a good diet maintains a balance between *yin* and *yang* foods. Food is also used therapeutically; hot *yang* foods (stronger, richer, spicier) are used for "cold" diseases (such as anemia, fatigue, and postpartum stress), and cold *yin* foods (low-calorie, bland foods such as vegetables and herbs) are taken to relieve "hot" diseases (such as measles, sore throats, irritability, and dry lips).

In the United States, we can now enjoy the unique cooking

styles and products of several regions of China—Mandarin, Hunan, Szechwan, Yunnan, and Cantonese—but the Asian diet here and in Asia is becoming more Americanized: higher in fat, protein, simple sugar, and cholesterol and lower in complex carbohydrates. Many Asians avoid dairy products, owing to a propensity for lactose intolerance. Desserts, which were once scarce, are becoming popular; and salt has superseded nonsodium alternatives, contributing to more hypertension.

In A/PI gerocounseling, conduct an in-depth interview to learn where each elder may be on the continuum of beliefs about food and health, because each person is different. Relate your interventions to your clients' beliefs, and connect any prescribed regimen to the rules of *yin* and *yang, fan* and *ts'ai,* so that your dietary advice is not in conflict with traditional cures.

At sites that provide meals—and in nursing homes—serve a rice dish with every meal for A/PI elders. You should know that chopsticks and a porcelain spoon for soup are still used by many older persons. Chinese etiquette requires young people to wait until elders begin to eat. The rice bowl is raised to the mouth.

Issues: Sources of Pain and Pride

A/PI immigrants brought traditional values that were admired by the dominant culture. Most immigrants and their children value academic excellence, hard work, strong family ties, filial piety, obedience, loyalty, good citizenship, and self-sacrifice and bringing honor (not shame) to ancestors. Such values have been expressed in behaviors that tend to result in lower rates of divorce, crime, drug and alcohol abuse, juvenile delinquency, and illegitimacy (though this is changing with increased acculturation).

It is not surprising that A/PIs are often called a "model minority"—the implication is that if one works hard enough, one can make it in the United States. However, this reasoning sometimes has been used to pit one minority against another, to exonerate mainstream society from guilt or from responsibility for the suffering of the poor, and to slacken efforts to provide needed services to A/PIs and others.

A/PI immigrants were confronted with massive prejudice, discrimination, and racism. During World War II, for example, thousands of loyal Japanese American citizens were placed in internment camps—almost like prisoners deprived of constitutional rights—without proof of guilt or benefit of the judicial process, is just one example.

Many A/PIs, underemployed and underpaid, were unwilling to tolerate conditions here and returned home. Others remained in A/PI ghettoes, believing that despite their life as a discriminated minority, the advantages of the host country outweighed the home country's disadvantages that included poverty, oppression, and sometimes physical danger. Still others rose in the professions and had a good income but nonetheless often experienced a "glass ceiling" at work, in the wider society, or both.

The list of those who "made it big" is long. To name a few is to leave out hundreds, but among the most notable are these:

Of Chinese ancestry: Anna May Wong, Hiram Fong, Dong Kingman, I.M. Pei, An Wang, Tsung Dao Lee, Chen Ning Yang, Betty Bao Lord, Amy Tan, Yo-Yo Ma, Maya Ying Lin, Michael Chang, Gary Locke, Connie Chung.

Of Japanese ancestry: D. T. Suzuki, Chiura Obata, Sessue Kintaro, Samuel Ichiye Hayakawa, Toshio Mori, Midori, Allen Say, Seiji Ozawa, and Kristi Yamaguchi.

Of Filipino ancestry: Pablo Manlapit, Carlos Bulosan, Phillip Vera Cruz, Bienvenido Santos, Jose Aruego, Fred Cordova, and Dorothy Cordova.

Of Hawaiian ancestry: Masayuki Massuaga, Daniel Inouye, Patsy Takemoto Mink, and Ellison Onizuka.

Of Korean ancestry: Younghill Kang, Chang-Ho Ahn, Phillip Ahn, Sammy Lee, K. W. Lee, Nam June Paik, and Myung-Whun Chung.

Of southeast Asian ancestry: Kith Pran, Luoth Yin, Eugene H. Trinh, and Andy Leonard.

Of Asian Indian ancestry: Dalip Singh Saund, Sirdar Jagjit Singh, and Zubin Mehta.

Still, the label "model minority" could be a form of reverse racism masking problems: poverty, overcrowding, poor health (the rate of tuberculosis among A/PIs is such as TB six times the national average), racism and discrimination, educational handicaps, lack of marketable skills, language barriers, daunting requirements for citizenship, and for students, culturally biased and irrelevant tests. Other things being equal, the Chinese, for example, have achieved less, not more, in the United States because of their race. Younger leaders are beginning to urge "polite, silent" Chinese elders to speak up.

EXERCISE

Think about the A/PI elders you met at the beginning of this part—Wen and Hulan Fu, Tony Mulos, Shon Young-Kim and Hwaja Kim, Mee Lee—and other A/PIs you know. How could any of the historical events listed at the beginning of this chapter have affected their lives, current problems, or cohorts?

Consider the dimensions of the Ethnic Lens: identity, demographics, immigration and migration experiences, cultural values, special issues. What part might each play in their present problems, beliefs, and attitudes?

Chapter 14

The A/PI Gero Chi Lens

In general, for Asian/Pacific Island elders successful acculturation has depended on ethnic values, identification with the homeland, experiences of immigration and relocation, education, social class, and facility with the native language and English. It has also depended on interactive factors in the Gero Chi Model: the self-system (particularly gender and spirituality); psychosocial development; how one has survived and is now aging in terms of biological, psychological, and social systems (especially social supports); and how the external environment interacts systemically with each factor. All play a role in the tasks of aging that must be accomplished for successful aging in any society.

The Self-System

The individual self-system, at the center of the Gero Chi Lens, is the basic unit—but when Dr. Owen Lum, a member of the Stanford Geriatric Education Center Core Faculty, was asked if it fit the Asian American elder, he thought not (personal communication, 1995). Lum suggested reducing the importance of the self-system in the Asian American model, because the extended family has more prominence. This observation is also reflected in the literature and will be our first adjustment entailed by the A/PI Ethnic Lens.

Self-Concept

A/PI elders tend to affiliate; the person may be seen not as individual in the western sense but as a locus of shared biographies: "The relationship defines the person, not vice versa" (Lieber, 1990, p. 72). A structural order in which everyone knows his or her place still allows for uniqueness, according to age, role, status, education, wealth, and wisdom (AARP, 1996). Lum (personal communication, 1997) wrote, "The self in Asian philosophy is tied to the past ("past heaven") and to the future ("future heaven"), with the *present* self [seen] as transitory."

Self-Esteem

In Asian societies where interdependence prevails, the individual comes second to the family; and individualism and independence—American values—are considered selfish, inconsiderate, or ungrateful. The Japanese use *enryo* (self-effacement) and indirect communication to describe the self. It is important to avoid disgrace, because it brings shame to the entire family, including ancestors.

Gender

As a result of the United States' immigration policies, the gender ratio among A/PI elders differs from that of other categories. In 1980, the overall ratio was 96 males to 100 females, in contrast to the general population, which had a ratio of 68 males to 100 females (Kii, 1984); and the ratio of men to women increases among older A/PIs. More A/PI women are married than comparable white women. This can be traced back to the A/PI bachelor societies, in which males outnumbered females.

The surplus of Korean females is an exception. Most of them are married; Korean men, it is reported, found American women too aggressive and disobedient and thus often returned to Korea for wives. Korean American women then, facing a shortage of men, acted accordingly. However, Korean Americans sometimes exaggerated their status and lifestyle in the United States when seeking a spouse; this frequently led to disappointments later (Locke, 1992).

Most A/PI older women defer to males, and the family hierarchy is patrilineal. Among Koreans, even when a husband abuses his wife, society protects the male—as is seen in the case of Shon Young-Kim and Hwaja. The eldest son is often the decision maker for an elder, and Hwaja's sons could not acknowledge that their father's violence was alcohol-related. In a marriage, roles are rigidly defined: The husband takes care of outside matters; the wife serves the husband and attends to family needs inside.

In contrast, Filipino women, usually more educated and powerful in their communities, have an equal role in controlling family matters, such as finances. Tony and Rose Bulos, for example, developed an amiable arrangement; he perceived himself as the patriarch of the family but she indirectly ran the show.

Spirituality

Asians have a long history of religious practices and beliefs based on seeking tranquillity and truth through the contemplation of nature. Elements of Taoism, Confucianism, Shamanism, and Buddhism often influence the everyday spirituality of even Christian A/PI elders. In Vietnam and in the Lees' home in Wisconsin, for example, the central room is a religious area, and family life and religious life are one.

Know the belief systems of your ethnogeroclients. These systems influence how clients view themselves, their afflictions, the world, you, and your services. You can use their beliefs benignly, to show your desire to understand and to help strengthen existing coping skills.

Confucianism, more a philosophy than a religion, directs practical problem solving in social, family, and governmental relationships; and the individual, deferring to the collective unit, is a part of and responsible to a series of related social positions. Harmony requires avoidance of conflict and a cheerful approach to all kinds of work. Ancestor worship and respect of peers are forms of moral and social control, and a whole village may laugh at a person who violates a social norm. In response to a question I raised at the Global Research Center for Health and Longevity in Bejing about elder abuse in China, I was told that it was handled successfully by "just village peer pressure" (personal communication, 1992).

Taoism, from the writings of Lao-Tzu, promises inner peace to those who will center their lives on the *dao* by contemplating nature. Taoist priests use elixirs along with traditional Chinese remedies to delay or prevent death. Shamanism, the major religion of northern Asia, believes in powerful spirits who can be influenced only by shamans. Buddhists believe that each person holds a seed of buddhahood, which is based on the "four noble truths":

1. There is a decadent village (truth of suffering).
2. There is a cause for this decadence (cause of suffering).
3. There is a hope that the village can be awakened (truth, hope for the cessation of suffering).
4. There is a way to awaken the village (truth of the method to extinguish the suffering).

One can reframe this metaphor of a village into a counseling model of beliefs about health and illness. In such a model, suffering ranges from physical and psychological pain to the insecurity of living in a transient world (Nakasone, 1990). Buddhahood (or health) is achieved by taking the "eightfold noble path": correct views of (1) understanding, (2) thought, (3) speech, (4) action, (5) livelihood, (6) exertion or endeavor, (7) mindfulness, and (8) right concentration or meditation.

Folk religion—with its many customs, beliefs, and fears regarding spirits and magical deities, including kitchen and earth gods—developed out of Buddhism and Taoism and is popular some among older A/PIs, such as Hulan Fu. Southeast Asians tend not to separate religion from everyday life, and many Cambodian and Laotian males spend a short time living as monks. Ninety percent of the Vietnamese adhere to a form of Buddhism or ancestor worship and believe in *karma*, a rebirth that is predetermined by good or bad deeds in one's previous life. After one has lived many worthy lives, liberation or spiritual release from the cycle of rebirth is achieved. Ancestors are worshiped for four generations; by the fifth generation, an ancestor has either been reborn or achieved heavenly bliss.

In America, many Chinese integrate the three Asian religions with Christianity. Koreans are often Methodist, Episcopalian, Catholic, or—like Shon and Hwaja Kim—members of the Church of Sun Myung Moon. Tony and Rose Bulos, like most Filipinos (and some Vietnamese), are Catholic. Some Asians are Muslims, or Christians belonging to Protestant sects.

Psychosocial Tasks

I found no specific applications of Erikson's model to A/PIs. But through interviews with A/PI providers—in particular, Dr. Owen Lum—and through various readings (Powell, 1983; Yamamoto and Iga, 1983; Yu & Kim 1983) I have developed some speculations about child rearing among traditional Asian Americans. These ideas provide clues about the personality development of A/PI elder clients and some intergenerational issues they may experience in extended families today. But I should point out that some American Asians give their children a traditional upbringing similar to their own, others blend eastern and western ways, and still others are totally acculturated—a warning against turning guarded generalizations into stereotypes. Asian American elders, like all elders, constitute a heterogeneous category, and there are many variations between and within various groups.

Hope (Trust versus Mistrust)

Asian parents give infants and toddlers unconditional regard and secure bonding. In Japan, mothering, a lifelong attachment, begins with long-term breast-feeding. In a comparative study, middle-class American mothers tended to leave infants alone but talked and stimulated them more; and the babies were more active, vocal, and playful. Japanese mothers were almost always with their babies and rocked and lulled them more to keep them contented. American mothers use baby bath tables while Japanese mothers take babies into the bathtub with them. Japanese babies are carried on the mother's back for the first year; children sleep with parents until age 10.

The sometimes overindulgent Korean mother pays exclusive attention to her newborn and, at first, visitors are not usually welcomed into the home—more for the sake of mother-infant togetherness than to avoid germs. Breast-feeding is felt to nourish the infant's body and pacify his or her rage. Wrapped in a shawl, babies are carried on the mother's back in their "piggy back years," ages 1 to 5; the movement is said to facilitate development of the nervous system. The American Korean working mother often brings her own mother over to be a built-in baby-sitter.

Practices differ among recent Vietnamese, Laos, and Hmong arrivals. Often, after a fatherless birth in a war-torn country, a mother and child endured traumatic evacuations and relocations that had dire effects on the child's development. Fathers who came to the United States, many who had been diagnosed with post traumatic stress disorder, often had low self-esteem also; they were frequently unemployed or underemployed while the mothers worked full time and this resulted in emotional and marital problems. Since severe physical punishment was allowed in their home countries, child abuse often occurred.

But usually, basic trust and a solid relationship develops during a carefully nurtured, prolonged infancy. This is not problematic in the later separation-individuation phase, because independence is not the Asian goal (Yu & Kim, 1983).

Will (Autonomy versus Shame)

"Here, Asians lose; shame and doubt results" (Lum, personal communication, 1995); "but" (on a more hopeful note) "they are positive attributes for children and society . . . shaping behavior early and helping the individual develop a necessary cautiousness."

Asian children are often toilet-trained early, sometimes before age 1. Korea, toilet-training is undemanding and casual; in fact, there are no words for it. But American Korean mothers report more demands and problems. In Japan, training is usually over by age 2, with no pressure. Likewise, infant sexuality and masturbatory behaviors go uncensured.

The Filipino family tends to be highly and vertically authoritative; good children obey their parents and older siblings and do not talk back or question. Discipline is firm and consists of physical punishment or shaming. Fathers discipline older children, usually sons. Grandparents, a secondary source of control, are often protective of grandchildren especially if a parent's punishment appears harsh. Traditional Filipino children kiss the hands of older family members in greeting and leave-taking; in this regard, American Filipino elders may complain about receiving less respect here—children do not address them as *manong* and *manang,* do not rise when an elder enters the room, and so on.

Japanese children are subjected to physical and emotional punishment; they maybe are pinched, laughed at, and threatened with being harmed by strangers. They may be locked outside the home in situations where an American child might be grounded or locked inside (Yamamoto & Iga, 1983, p. 173).

Purpose (Initiative versus Guilt)

In Korean families, disciplinary tactics that overemphasize obedience and conformity can hinder self-reliance; also shame and disgrace, reinforced by a fear of shaming ancestors, may foster a need for acceptance and sensitivity to disapproval.

Although unconditional love and indulgence tend to be the pattern during early childhood, this changes abruptly when a child starts school and is held to strict expectations. Lum feels that this sudden change reflects a rigidly obsessive-compulsive cultural system and notes that while there are few individual diagnoses of obsessive-compulsiveness or separation anxiety, phobias, excessive rumination, somatic concerns, and guilt are seen in cases of depression.

In Korea, parents' indulgence typically switches to prohibitions when a child reaches age 6. Strict rules and moral codes are introduced—at first gently, later firmly. Filial respect and ancestor worship are imposed early; the family is considered the most important symbol in life, and its preservation is an important duty. "Confucian ideas and centuries-old cultural conditioning produced a social system with the pattern of submission of the individual to the family, of the young to the old, and of woman to man" (Yu & Kim, 1983, p. 150).

Among Asians, the oedipal conflict does not get played out intensely until adolescence. Reasons given are the characteristics of the extended family and the fact that in early child care, the male versus female model is not well defined. Both parents participate in parenting. Even Korean fathers, who traditionally thought of parenting as unmasculine, are more active parents in America— their more liberated Korean wives insist on it. Korean children also sleep in their parents' room but seem to show no evidence of psychosexual problems. The Japanese boy is not expected to grow beyond the oedipal situation but rather should develop a masculine identity while still attached to the mother (Yamamoto & Iga, 1983, p. 171).

Competence (Industry versus Inferiority)

Asian children must imitate their parents' initiative and be industrious but should also be humble about their achievements. Even a child who gets A's may have feelings of doubt and inferiority. "The Asian child," said Lum, (1995), "tends to compare [the] self to an unreachable goal."

School is usually very important to Filipinos, and to other A/PIs. It is considered a way out of poverty—a passport to jobs, economic security, and social acceptance. Parents heavily go into debt for the eldest child's education; then that child is expected to help younger siblings. This is called "debt of gratitude," and "ungrateful" children become outcasts .

Korean children are often under much pressure to achieve academically and to be admitted to elite high schools and colleges; and they must study long hours or face the severe trauma of failure. Most younger American Korean children function well in school, social relationships, and cognitive competition. But others, owing to culture shock at school and teasing by peers, report diminished self-esteem; they may consider their Asian features ugly, inferior, or shameful. This problem is often resolved by age 7; but in some cases it continues, affecting personality, functioning, or adjustment (Yu & Kim, 1983).

Fidelity (Identity versus Diffusion)

Culture and ethnicity affect the quest for identity, which is played out in different ways. For example, because of recent turmoil, identity is more of a problem in Vietnamese society; other Asians, from strict and stable family structures, knew their place in family, society, and government, and there was no question about belonging. This is, of course, different for Asian immigrants to the United States and their offspring, who may suffer from lifelong identity problems, depending on the speed of acculturation and its different degrees within a family. It appears that the faster the acculturation takes place, the greater the stress due to separation from the extended family.

Identity conflicts are seen, for instance, when Korean adolescents want to be more like American teens and their elders want them to keep traditional values. "In this connection," wrote Yu and

Kim (1983), "Korean youths are faced with a double dilemma: the absence of belonging to a vital and nourishing milieu of contemporary American society, and a sense of disconnectedness with their own original ethnic heritage" (p. 155). These authors explored three patterns of identity formation that might also fit Korean American elders:

1. *Full Korean identity.* They just live here.
2. *Korean-American identity.* Considering themselves to be fully assimilated or acculturated, they strive to keep positive values of both cultures. While they risk becoming marginalized, they appear most energized, motivated, and adaptive.
3. *Full American identity.* They deny and are dissociated from fellow Koreans and their values in order to become "all American."

Sexual issues also become important in adolescence. Filipino families tend to be very strict with adolescents, providing little sex education—which must therefore be acquired elsewhere, from peers. Public displays of affection are considered vulgar, and dating is supposed to relate to marriage. Females are expected to maintain a good reputation, and males are expected to avoid having to get married and thus having to forgo education and career plans. Matchmaking is still common. In a culture that places much stress on loyalty, casual dating is uncommon because the breakup of a romance can be severely stressful to young people.

Love (Intimacy versus Isolation)

"This gets played out differently for Asians," Lum said. "There is no isolation of self in the identity with the cultural group. The cost to the individual is the loss of intimacy and initiative." The Asian, like others, wants intimacy but can suffer from intimacy—perhaps because of a need to keep an emotional distance in an enmeshed family in a crowded apartment on a crowded continent. In Japan, I saw "love hotels" where Japanese couples could escape from their crowded conditions for a few hours of intimacy. Because many Asians are used to such crowding, one wonders if Asian elders have fewer problems adjusting to, say, a double room in a nursing home.

Belonging is an important Japanese value; the focus is on collectiveness and group cooperation. Being tied to groups—the family, the school, and the company—is how one identifies oneself, thus eliminating the need for much verbal communication. A glib person is suspect and likely to be considered dishonest; individuals learn to internalize or somatize problems rather than act out.

Care (Generativity versus Stagnation)

Generativity is greatly valued in these interdependent societies where duty, responsibility, and loyalty are so important. Asian American immigrant elders have often struggled for family survival and to offer their children opportunities in the United States.

Wisdom (Integrity versus Despair)

Lum said that traditionally, there is almost a liberation from responsibility after age 60. Growing older was a time to put one's life work aside, with cultural "permission" to pursue fulfillment in other ways, such as enhanced spirituality and health, the arts, and calligraphy. I did observe this in my tours of senior centers and nursing homes in Bejing in 1992. But I speculated that this may change because Asians are living longer and the "young-old" are sandwiched between generations, with responsibilities for the "old-old" and for their grandchildren. Here in the United States, as in China, much of the responsibility for child care rests with many A/PI elders. Some service providers I interviewed said that this almost bordered on elder abuse.

Do such conditions lead to integrity or despair? "Despair," wrote Lum (personal communication, 1997), "means the loss of the cultural promise of integral blending with the whole." Many A/PI elders continue to be useful—or used—in the "whole community." The despair noted by some observers has to do with the fact that many of the expectations about being honored in old age are not realized in the United States as Asian families become more Americanized. Ego integrity is achieved not for the self but for the family group, in the passing on of the culture to the next generation. Lum believed that Asian elders are still highly valued and had few problems here.

The Subset Systems

The A/PI Ethnic Lens continues to imply changes in the Gero Chi Model as we consider biopsychosocial systems of elderly A/PIs and their families.

The Biological System

Along with skin color, small stature, and eye shape (which makes cataract surgery more difficult), Asians have physiologic differences that affect their sensitivity to certain medications. Tien (1984) warned that they require lower dosages and experience more side effects from even low to medium doses of some medicines.

Health Status

Available data are meager. A/PIs' life expectancy is greater than that of whites, and they suffer less from the major diseases (Liu & Yu, 1985). But A/PIs have higher A/PI rates of tuberculosis, hepatitis, anemia, and hypertension; and Japanese and Chinese American elders have more multi-infarct dementia and osteoporosis than the general population (Hasegawa, 1989). The Fus—in our examples at the beginning of this part—fit this profile: Hulan suffers from severe osteoporosis and Wen died of a stroke resulting from hypertension. Tony Mulos, too, suffers from hypertension.

A/PIs superior health status is attributed to their diet—lower in fat and higher in carbohydrates—and to their lower rates of obesity; but increased artery disease is seen with Americanization. There are wide differences among groups, and the positive statistics may reflect only the healthy Asian majority. Health also varies with time of immigration; recent immigrants and refugees often have poor health—they especially incur heart disease, cancer, diabetes, and accidents—and death rates are higher among the foreign-born.

Health Beliefs

Again, these differ; some among A/PIs have completely adopted the western medical model; some adhere to eastern ways; and some straddle both cultures. Such differences affect prevention, compliance, use of advance directives, and the overall success of your work. Because family takes precedence over self, it is the family, most often the eldest son, who makes decisions about health care; but you must know how each family makes such decisions.

Asian elderly people may be likely to consult practitioners of traditional eastern medicine for sprains, puncture wounds, internal bleeding, arthritis, earaches, and headaches, high blood pressure, stroke, and general internal pain—and when western medicine doesn't bring a cure. Many expect eastern medicine to replenish the blood's active energy, tranquilize the mind, and relieve muscle spasms. Usually they see a western practitioner for surgery, broken bones, and infectious diseases.

Adherents of Chinese medicine from China, Korea, Japan, Indochina, and the Philippines believe that health is a balance between opposites: *yin* (cold, moist, passive, dark, female) and *yang* (hot, dry, forceful, light, male). In illness (an imbalance), the vital force (*chi*) is out of harmony and not properly circulating, so efforts (acupuncture, acupressure, herbal remedies) are directed toward restoring balance.

The Vietnamese believe that illness is caused by imbalance, spirits, or "wind" illnesses. In one case, abuse was suspected when an elder had distinctive stripes and circles on his back—which were actually a result of "coining and cupping," superficial dermal treatments to release excess heat or wind. Some Vietnamese believe that surgery dishonors ancestors because the physical body belongs to them. Hmongs fear this offense will cause loss of soul (mental illness). Nguyen (1989) reported that Vietnamese elders often do not use medications properly, stopping when they feel better and saving some for the "next time." Many believe that western medicines are inappropriate for the Asian body and cite side effects and costs.

Combining western medicine (considered *yang*) with Chinese medical practices (*yin*) is common. For example, a person may bathe or take medicine only in cold water or take half of a prescription. Herbal teas, soups, or poultices are sometimes substituted for food. Some patients may refuse surgery or a blood test, fearing that it will reduce the supply of blood and *chi* (Yeo, 1995). Hulan Fu's inconsistent medical compliance has been a constant source of frustration to her in doctors Boston, for example.

The Psychological System

Mental Health Beliefs

Are A/PI elders different from whites as regards personality? Here, cultural values can shed light, as culture, through the family, is a chief sculptor of personality. Important to personality development among many A/PIs are family obligations and reciprocity, obedience to rules and roles, a sense of fatalism, filial piety, *enryo* (self-effacement). To Filipinos and others, important values include *hiya* (shame) and respect for authority; to Koreans, *che myun* (face-saving), harmonious relations, and preservation of family honor; to Hawaiians, *aloha* (Browne & Broderick, 1994).

An individual's spiritual philosophy also guides the personality. Buddhists, usually pessimistic and fatalistic, stress harmony, self-discipline, humility, and following the middle path. Confucians respect elders, hierarchial rank, and loyalty; loss of face, or shame, keeps society moral. Taoists solve problems by taking an indirect approach; they avoid confrontation and practice patience and simplicity. The Vietnamese, believing that life is brief, often see the individual as insignificant and stress denial of self-gratification, control of emotions, avoidance of impulsive behavior, and promotion of nonconfronting, harmonious situations.

Mental Health Status

Do A/PI elders have a high degree of life satisfaction? High suicide rates may indicate that they do not. Suicide is more prevalent among A/PI elders than any other category of elderly Americans. The suicide rate among Chinese women age 65–74, is three times higher than among comparable whites; for Chinese women age 75–80 years (many 'picture brides'), it is seven times higher (Liu & Yu, 1985).

Kim (1990) relates these figures to incongruities between Asian values and American realities and to the fact that suicide is acceptable to Buddhists—as may be shown by the high rates also found among the Japanese, Vietnamese, Hmong, and others. Koreans and Thais condone suicide as a ways to shed the shame incurred from ancestors. Suicides among first-generation Chinese American women who were brought here as "picture brides" were attributed to isolation and "despair for their poor health and inability to obtain satisfactory medical care (Liu & Yu, 1985, p. 48). The relatives of Hulan Fu, one of our case examples, fear that she will commit suicide if she is sent to a nursing home.

Suicide appears to be sensitive to culture and acculturation. The longer ago an Asian American's immigration took place, the lower the risk of suicide. Highest risks are found among the less educated, the poor, and Buddhists.

Japanese males and other A/PIs tend to be hospitalized more for schizophrenia than for other mental illnesses; but is this a reality or a habitual classification made by biased diagnosticians? Affective diseases such as recurrent depression and unipolar disorders are underreported. Since to many Asians mental illness is an unacceptable illness, it often goes untreated and hence unreported, as in the case of Tony Mulos's long-term depression.

Comparisons between Chinese American and American nursing homes showed a prevalence of multi-infarct dementia four to six times greater than Alzheimer's dementia. A study in Shanghai related both cognitive impairment and Alzheimer's disease to being female and uneducated (Morioka-Douglas & Yeo, 1990). Some A/PI families attribute dementia to "old age"; Mee Lee's family, for instance, thought her confusion and combativeness were due to "strong personality and meanness."

Among the Chinese, there are three culture-bound syndromes related to brief psychosis: *koro* (a dramatic and threatening sense of panic that the penis will shrink into the abdomen with resultant death); *frigophobia* (an excessive fear and intolerance of cold in ambient temperature and food); and *shen-k'uei weakness* (fatigue, insomnia, anxiety, and hypochondriasis related to sexual problems, panic, or anxiety disorders).

Drug abuse is sometimes seen among A/PI elders. It may take the form of using someone else's medicine or of using opium and other depressive hallucinogenics sanctioned by many first-generation Koreans, Chinese, Hmong, and Cambodians. Rates of alcoholism are low, but—as with Mr. Kim—alcoholism does exist. For the Chinese, alcoholism has never been a social or medical problem, probably because they have a high sensitivity to alcohol and because traditional Chinese society prevents alcohol abuse with strong social controls. With increased westernization here and in Hong Kong and Taiwan, increases in alcoholism are seen (Lin, 1983).

The Sociological System

Aspects of A/PI sociological systems have been covered through-out this section. The interdependent, extended, rigid family sys-tem, held in highest esteem, is the primary social unit in most southeast Asian cultures where the family clan rates highest. Filial piety and honor to the aged are strong influences, complemented by other values: obligation, reciprocity, and obedience to roles and rules.

Rules regarding relationships between family members and non-relatives are many. Among the Vietnamese, respect for more knowl-edgeable or elderly persons is essential and is expressed through prescribed appropriate body movements. One bows one's head to a respected elder. Hands clasped at the chest signify a greeting. Both hands are used to pass an object; women do not shake hands; only the elderly may touch another person's head in public (and then only a child's); the only accepted beckoning gesture is to use the entire hand with fingers upward for persons or down-ward for animals. Kissing in public is taboo.

Caregiving is almost always provided by the family or clan unless that is impossible, and a nursing home is the last alterna-tive. As with Hulan Fu, a case manager will probably seek out grandnieces and grandnephews to see if someone will take an elder in. Even in Sacramento's Asian Community Nursing Home, Asians, like other ethnic elders, are underrepresented, although there are ethnic foods, programs, and cultural and religious activ-ities; ethnic volunteers; and an "ethnic-competent" staff.

Hara (personal communication, 1995) noted a recent increase in Asian nursing home residents, and Yang (personal communication, 1997) said that more Hmong elders are now living independently. Such trends are related to the fact that more women (the usual caregivers) are in the workforce, elders are living longer and thus have more long-term needs, and American housing does not lend itself to large extended families. While Mee Lee and her husband preferred living with their family, the small apartment would not contain them all, and they had to get HUD housing.

So despite the primacy of family, the many-generation home is often not a reality for A/PIs. Even in Bejing, a study found that more Chinese elders, like their American counterparts, wanted to live near but not with their adult children— experiencing "intimacy at a distance." In 1992 I visited independent senior housing apartments in Bejing with the American Society on Aging (ASA) and found them to be plainer but much like those in the United States, complete with senior activity centers, some community health facilities, and sports complexes (Burlingame, 1992).

A/PI elders tend to live with their children in cases of extreme poverty, ill health, or language difficulties, or when they are needed as baby-sitters. Many Koreans proudly regard separate-generation living as a way to promote their children's success and happiness. For many A/PIs, Chinatowns, Manilatowns, and Japantowns became forms of extended families; and Asian American associations sponsoring mutual aid arose, such as the Chinese tongs, Japanese benefit associations, and communal associations within Asian Christian churches and Buddhist temples. Similarly, ethnic-sensitive health services such as the On Lok model moved into these communities, reinforcing the sense of extended family.

But as with the "model majority" concept, the Asian family is not in place for everyone. Widowed and childless, 93-year-old Hulan Fu finds herself increasingly frail and with little family support.

Practices related to death and dying vary from family to family owing to different religious and spiritual traditions, different environments, and different degrees of acculturation. Beliefs and practices about death and dying are usually a mix.

Asians often talk about a "good death"—dying peaceably in old age surrounded by family. A hospital is considered a peaceful place to die, not a place to get well. A "bad death" occurs when a family thinks a patient is not strong enough for the cultural role of longevity and therefore insists on aggressive interventions to prolong life. The Global Resource Center for Health and Longevity in Bejing, a governmental agency that hosted my ASA trip in 1992, aims for a life of 100 years for each Chinese citizen in the near future (Burlingame, 1992).

The System of Aging Tasks

A/PI elders have the same tasks of aging as all other American elders. A ninth task—preservation of ethnic roots in harmony with an American identity—can be added.

EXERCISE

Think again of the case examples at the beginning of this part. After layering the A/PI Ethnic Lens onto the Gero Chi Lens, what information about A/PI elders do you now have that adds to a deeper understanding of these A/PI elders and their families, and other A/PI elders that you know? What more do you need to know?

Chapter 15

A/PIs and Gerocounseling

Throughout these chapters, we have seen that the Ethnic Lens for each category implies substantial changes in how we must view our ethnogeroclients. Likewise, a new cultural sensitivity should also alter how counseling can be done. Let us now apply the Ethnic Lens to the A/PI Gerocounseling Model to learn what changes should be considered.

Generic Gerocounseling

Ethics Skills

Many A/PIs prefer that health care providers talk to family or clan members rather than the patient about medical matters. Some believe that a sick person should be protected, like a child. Some feel that telling a patient he or she is terminally ill destroys hope and can hasten or even cause death. Some feel that openly acknowledging the gravity of a situation implies that the health professional has given up hope.

Again, you must be aware of differences in cultural beliefs and practices regarding health care, among and within families. Each family member may be at a different place in the continuum of beliefs about health; and this can create barriers to problem solving and the use of services. Conflicts can arise when an A/PI elder wants to practice traditional Chinese medicine but younger family members want western care.

With elders of the dominant culture, your goal is typically to help them maintain autonomy and independence; but your work with A/PI clients might involve helping them achieve an important A/PI value, family harmony instead.

When the family is the client, you may find yourself confiding information to a specified family member, not to the elder. You will need to identify this person immediately so that the elder can sign the necessary consent forms for release of information. This bicultural process will show your desire to work with an existing family system, and it will protect you. In some systems, the eldest son will make the important decisions; among the Hmong, it may be the clan leader. Sometime the designated person is the one with the greatest facility in English.

Relationship Skills

Counselors have countertransference, feelings, and attitudes from our past that are evoked in current ethnogerocounseling. This is best managed by knowing ourselves, including our own ethnic roots, as discussed in Chapter 1.

Likewise, clients bring transference, feelings, and attitudes to our relationship; we can manage these by knowing about a client's cohort, culture, social class, and immigration history.

Many A/PI elders were not socialized to express feelings, to be direct, or to disclose personal matters. For many, there is a legacy of distrust of institutions and bureaucrats, based on painful experiences of immigration and migration. Many do not understand counseling or psychology, do not accept any deviation from the norm, feel shame about needing help, or feel that they have shamed their families and ancestors. Because of these barriers, when they do come for any form of assistance, it is likely to be for more serious problems. Also, those born in the United States and those who have been here a long time are more likely than recent arrivals to seek help for personal matters. Don't take resistant behaviors personally, but try to find ways to make the geroclient feel more comfortable.

Trust will be a big issue. Yeung (personal communication, 1955) said that pride or ("face") is often an initial impediment to building a relationship. Most A/PIs feel shame about having a psychological problem, seeing it as an admission of personal or family wrongdoing, or even as a punishment. They may rather talk about bodily symptoms so as to "save face," so that is where you will often have to begin. Tony Mulos's case manager never used the word, *depression* or *antidepressant* to Tony; that would have upset him. Tony took his medication for "energy."

Huang (personal communication, 1995) said that in order to not loose face, a client will often not tell you the real problem; you must infer it. For instance, a client may not get along with her daughter-in-law but may not want anyone to know. At her senior center, she tells everyone how wonderful she the daughter-in-law is, but that is untrue. Huang advised against confronting the client in such a situation, but a home visit may help, indirectly, to bring the issue to the surface. As the counselor visits the home and becomes less of a stranger and more like "family," talking about a problem may become easier. Share some casual facts about yourself. Since some A/PIs share personal information only with family, your sharing makes it easier for them to share with you.

While some A/PI clients may deny reality or suppress feelings, others tend to somatize as a way of defending themselves against an admission of mental illness. Depression, for instance, may be described as constipation, headaches, or apathy, and the client may wish to start with concrete explanations and remedies. Taking too much social history and asking psychological questions at intake may lead some clients to believe you think they lack self-discipline, are lazy, have character flaws, or come from a "bad family." The client may become defensive, may withhold information, and may not return.

But a counselor's detachment may not be effective either. Many A/PI clients need reassurance that they are okay and that confidentiality will be maintained.

Since some A/PI elders are unsophisticated with regard to counseling, what might they desire? I was told that usually they expect an authoritative person who will not talk much but will solve problems and make the symptoms go away by giving advice or a prescription. Clients often want structured, focused sessions and concrete information about the counseling process, its goals, the nature of the counseling relationship, and what to expect. They need an explanation of why a clinical history is important (if it is), why you need to know about previous treatment, and why family background and a list of psychosocial stressors are discussed. Such an explanation, along with nonjudgmental, nonthreatening questions, can reassure clients that you do not see a problem as a character flaw. This can be a difficult process with a sensitive client, but using this pragmatic problem-solving approach will pay off.

Other forms of transference will affect how the client treats you. Some may respond to you with Filipino *pakikisama*, courtesy and willingness to go along to gain approval of someone in authority. Others may treat you like someone powerful in an analogous (though very different) position in the home country. Others may go along with everything you say out of courtesy but may have no intention of following your suggestions.

I asked A/PI counselors for tips. They recommended engaging in personal dialogue before discussing a problem, offering environmental and practical help, making home visits, being available at irregular hours, offering telephone sessions, not doing paperwork in front of a client, and making collateral contacts, with the permission of client *and* family.

McBride (personal communication, 1995) said attention to gender issues is important. The sex of the counselor should be considered in assigning cases and discussed in the counseling itself. Many A/PIs feel uncomfortable about discussing certain matters with the opposite sex—or with someone younger. If your background is different from the client's, discuss what it means and feels to be from a certain group.

In a recent survey, A/PI elders said they expected "respectful behavior" from health care providers. But respect can differ from culture to culture. With many Asians, for example, it is respectful to ask permission to take a history, give a physical exam, or take blood. For many Vietnamese, respect means not raising one's voice, not touching an elder's head (where the soul resides), and not beckoning an elder with upturned crooked fingers.

To many, reciprocity is important in a relationship and necessary to self-esteem. The Filipino client may want to give a gift to the provider, to avoid shame and indebtedness. At first, Pete refused Tony and Rose Mulos's invitations to stay for supper because he was trained not to socialize with clients. But when he realized that his refusals were hurting more than helping, he accepted.

Be careful not to read pathology into relationship patterns that are appropriate in a particular culture. A client who is turning to you for expert advice may appear overly dependent but may in reality be problem-solving. A client's unusual interest in your life may seem suspicious but may simply reflect a strongly affiliative culture. When elders praise or advise you, that may simply be the role elders play in their society, so do not automatically regard such behavior as a violation of professional boundaries or neurotic transference. Instead, see it—and use it positively—as gracious-ness, charm, and acceptance.

The idea that A/PIs are difficult to engage in counseling is a myth. Tsui and Schultz (1985) said that high underutilization and drop out rates are common but asked whether this could be due to counselors' unfamiliarity with salient cultural issues. They warned against misunderstanding cues that arise from a culture that em-phasizes deference to authority, strong family bonds, well-defined social roles and expectations, communal responsibilities, and a pragmatic view of life and personal relationships (p. 561). All these factors can influence a client's or a family's transference.

There is no question that, other things being equal, those who know the culture and language will be most successful with ethnic people. Skalland (personal communication, 1995) told about a group of 25 to 30 Korean American elders who met in a small park shelter affiliated with her senior center and apartments. Most had been living there for ten years, but few spoke English, and they came as a group and did not mix. When asked for feedback, they always responded, "Everything is fine." Their group leader was Korean too, and she taught them English and line dancing. When she left several years ago, the group members stopped coming. When she came back, they did too.

"Given the interpersonal complexity of traditional cultures, es-tablishing relationships that mirror those found in family groups or in friendship networks may be helpful to the client as a means of guiding the interpersonal process with the counselor" (Ishisaka & Takagi, 1982, p. 155). These authors suggested that the counselor match the client's manners and charm, ask about the client's health, offer a cup of tea, suggest that the client take off his or her coat, offer a comfortable chair, and accept a thank-you gift or praise. If you are invited to a family gathering or given referrals, accept them gracefully as the client's desire to express gratitude. All such responses indicate concern and caring.

Communication Skills

The following suggestions from people who work with A/PIs may start you on your way to becoming culturally sensitive in your communication with A/PI elders.

Speak in quiet tones to show respect and caring. Generalize about feelings other people from a particular group have while still indicating that each client is unique. Use positive general "feelers" such as, "It must take a lot of patience to cope with such a hard situation," instead of direct intrusive questions such as, "How do you cope with the problem?"

Clients who are vague or who circumvent the issue may be testing your attitude. Don't express surprise, distaste, or impatience; avoid probing deeply, since this may be seen as rude and intrusive. Hulan Fu did not always level with her case manager because after having waited so long to immigrate to the United States, she was fearful that anything she revealed might cause her to be to sent back. To gain your approval, clients' may tell you what they think you want to hear. If they do, reframe this as fear or courtesy.

Certain subjects must be handled delicately in most A/PI cultures. Also, confrontations may be unacceptable as they tend to be among Filipinos and Chinese. Often a family will use a go-between to solve interpersonal problems. A doctor, instead of a family member, may be the one to say, "You need a nursing home." Lum (personal communication, 1995) suggested using an intermediary, usually a distant family member, to advocate or help speak for a passive relative rather than urge behaviors that are foreign and alien to the culture.

Learn at least a few common words in your client's language. In Filipino culture (which values patience and tact), there are many terms that reveal guidelines for communication. A person who must be *pakikisama* will say, "*Siguro nga,*" which means "I guess so," in order to rule out disagreement. Failure to express gratitude or to reciprocate would be to deny *utang na loob*.

The Japanese too have special courtesies of communication.

Japanese clients will consider you rude if you comment on how well they speak English, if you chew gum, or if you eat standing up. Avoid physical contact and looking directly in another person's eyes. Don't assume that a nod or a smile indicates agreement or even understanding. A Japanese person may say yes several times before giving you a straight answer, so ask if the client has understood what you said. "Okay" means "no" and *san* at the end of a person's name signifies respect.

Hara (personal communication, 1995) reported that at the Asian Community Nursing Home in Sacramento, California common words used for personal communication among A/PI residents were taught to the entire staff as part of in-service training. Learn your clients' special words and terms, and learn to use them properly.

Assessment

We have stressed that in making assessments and planning interventions, it is important to learn about your clients' belief or meaning systems. While some older clients may see themselves as victims of traumatic events, others offer moral explanations, seeing their problems as a punishment for moral failures or violations of culturally prescribed conduct. A Chinese client may attribute suffering to a lack of filial piety; a Japanese may consider it cosmic retribution for misbehavior; a Filipino Christian may believe that personal grief, misfortune, or mental illness is a consequence of unexpiated sins.

Physical Assessments

Yeo (1995) wrote that practitioners of Chinese medicine and Korean *hanbang* do not use laboratory tests or extensive exams; thus the Chinese American and Korean elders may not understand why we insist on including them. Many clients are embarrassed by genitourinary issues, ailments, and examinations and expect to be asked beforehand whether or not they want such testing.

Psychological Assessments

Paper-and-pencil tests are sometimes inappropriate for A/PIs, who may prefer immediate feedback on each question. Obviously, the

Mini-Mental State Examination (MMS) and similar tests of cognition would include items irrelevant for new immigrants and would need revision to ensure validity.

The Minnesota Multiphasic Personality Inventory (MMPI) may also be questionable as a diagnostic tool for A/PI elders. It predicts suicide fairly well with non-Asians because it measures a respondent's energy level; but is not a good predictor for Asians, who often talk negatively about it (Lum, 1993).

The Geriatric Depression Scale (Yesavage et al., 1983), a favorite instrument for elders of the dominant culture, is not often used with Asians, because it does not ask enough questions about psychosomatic factors and because Asians tend to somatize depression. But high scores on the Zung and Beck Inventories usually reflect a high degree of somatization and also existential concerns about trying to adapt to American lifestyles (Lum, 1993, p. 44). Because of somatization in depression among Asian Americans, there may be secondary gains from being a patient.

Family Assessments

Because many Asians tend to be unexpressive, one should look for nonverbal behaviors; videotaping a session can help in family assessment. Look for nonverbal clues to excessively enmeshed relationships, distorted boundaries, patterns of dependency, and latent themes. Also, listen carefully to understand whom they are discussing; it may be an ancestor who consumes them with obligation and guilt.

Clinical Interview Assessments

In ethnogerocounseling, as in the assessment of all elders, the findings of the clinical interview are often the most reliable, but even they are subject to the assessor's skill and biases. Gerocounselors have their own ethnic lenses, and countertransference may interfere with assessments.

For example, affective disorders are often underreported among Chinese Americans whereas schizophrenia and manic depression may be over-diagnosed (Lum, 1993). In a study of 10 white and Chinese American therapists who assessed white and Chinese clients in videotaped interviews, the white therapists saw the white clients as affectionate, adventurous, and capable; the Chinese therapists saw them as active, aggressive, and rebellious. Chinese American therapists saw Chinese American clients as adaptable, alert, dependable, friendly, and practical; white therapists saw them as anxious, awkward, confused, nervous, quiet, and reserved (Lum, 1993). Tseng, McDermott, and Maretzski (1974) devised a manual to help mental health workers elicit and understand such variables of ethnic behaviors.

Ethnogerocounseling Modalities

Psychotherapy has not been widely used in Asia, and this leads many to think that it is ineffective with Asians. In China, there is much resistance to insight-oriented psychotherapy, which appears to run counter to Chinese thinking:

1. The Chinese seek harmonious interpersonal relations and looking inward is not considered a solution.
2. Issues of sex and intimacy are not discussed with strangers.
3. Mental illness is believed to be organic, not conflict-ridden.
4. Communication is nonverbal and symbolic. (Lin, 1983)

Western psychiatric treatments such as psychotropic drugs, electroconvulsive therapy, and insulin shock therapy are widely used in Asia, but there is little research on their effectiveness there. Antidepressants often do not fit in well with A/PIs physiology and habits: patients tend to require lower dosages, and they frequently take an antidepressant only as needed, discontinuing it when they feel better. The Vietnamese prefer injections.

Family therapy is the treatment of choice for most A/PIs because of the organic nature of Asian families and the integral role each member plays within the family system; but harmony—not individuation—is the goal.

Many A/PIs find *group therapy* traumatic because even sharing one to one is hard enough. A group that requires some verbal aggression may demand too much emotional effort from Asians and be culturally dystonic. For Japanese clients, Kaneshige (1973) recommended:

1. A nonthreatening climate encourages verbal communication.
2. Members' listening skills should be encouraged.
3. Nonexpressive sharing should not be interrupted.
4. The leader ensures confidentiality, clarifies, interprets expressions, challenges criticisms, and recognizes authority roles.
5. The leader verbalizes the group's differences in cultural value.
6. The goal is personal growth, not denial of ethnic identity.

Ethnogerocounseling Interventions

Chapter 3 discussed some important principles for interventions in gerocounseling, such as environmental press, parsimony, values, individual learning styles, gentleness, and a systems outlook. The A/PI Ethnic Lens stresses two more: ethnic sensitivity and empowerment.

Ethnic Sensitivity

Ethnic sensitivity has been stressed throughout this book. It includes countless little—though not trivial—commonplace ways. Asking a simple question about your client's ethnic culture shows your desire to understand. Some areas are:

Food

When serving food in a day treatment center, a senior center, or a nursing home, offer rice with each meal. In the United States, Asian Americans' diet has tended to become less healthful because of an overabundance of meat here and the high cost of vegetables. A/PI elders may need education—in their own language—about avoiding animal fats, avoiding too much meat, and returning to vegetables.

Language

Offer professional translation services for the major language groups and teach key words to non-Asian staff members. Print newsletters, activity schedules, and ads in major languages, and use language resources to teach elders and their families about patients' rights, power of attorney, informed consent, the nature of illnesses, and treatments.

Literacy

Do not assume that an A/PI client can read English or his or her own native language; often, a video is preferable to print. The Wisconsin Geriatric Education Center, for example, created a video explaining the Patient Self-Determination Act and advance directives for Hmong clients in their language.

Staff Training

Train the staff to be culturally sensitive and competent. Teach beliefs, behaviors, and explanatory health models and use them in care plans. Assess religious practices. When possible, for instance, include a shaman or another religious healer if a client still believes in anamism. Get help. Use trained, trusted translators, consultants, colleagues, and mentors from your clients' ethnic groups.

Mary O'Brien's frustration over her inability to help Mee Lee's family led her to find a Hmong consultant, who advised Mary to work within the existing family and clan structure. Respite and day care were vital to Mee's safety and Kia's health, but, she asked, could they be organized and obtained *within* the family? The Hmong mentor advised that instead of offering too much help and "invading the family," Mary help by being first a social friend and a comforting listener. In general, he advised, don't do paper work in front of a family, and stay away from the subject of death.

Yang (personal communication, 1997) said that if a nursing home is needed, the extended family should be involved in the decision and in the plan, so that the burden does not fall on only one family member.

Personal Empowerment

Begin ethnic-sensitive counseling with what Lum called "belief therapy." He helps clients to be comfortable with their own identity, resolve cultural conflicts, and reinforce what is solid and good. "Western counselors often have trouble with Asian shame. It is close to the superego and strong; one cannot make an Asian shameless," he said. "Work with it; don't try to erase it."

I wondered how an Asian lives with shame without making amends. Lum helps the client to ventilate (if possible), to grieve, and to probe for existential issues. Is it possible to make a shameful deed or shameful feelings heroic? If not, one can work within cultural values:

1. Use concepts of shame or fate in stories or metaphors as explanations and to inspire growth.
2. Be aware that understatement and indirection can express powerful emotions, such as grief or anxiety.
3. Expect conflict and confusion regarding identity and norms.
4. Don't try to change ritualized self-depreciation; it is a way of emphasizing the primacy of the group over the individual.
5. Reinforce willingness to endure and persevere while suffering.
6. Deal delicately with taboo subjects such as alcoholism, family violence, finances, and violations of sexual norms. Reframe taboos, seeing them not as psychological denial but as family loyalty.
7. Be aware that traditional events, such as seeing deceased ancestors, are metaphorical, not delusional.
8. Venting may be inappropriate; many Asians highly regard a thoughtful silence or a brief insightful comment.

Environmental Empowerment

Skalland, who is a director of a senior housing facility, noted overt as well as subtle forms of elder abuse that go unreported. In some areas, it is common to lock up an elder in a small apartment for 10 hours a day to care for small children. Skalland has found Mandarin Chinese to be especially overprotective and isolating. Many elders have saved money to come here, have given what is left to their adult children, and now see themselves as "cheap baby-sitters." While this is not what they expected, they are too ashamed to admit that they are being abused.

One constructive arrangement is to let such grandparents bring their grandchildren to activities at a senior center. They bring food for the children or take the meal the center provides outside to share with the children. Another constructive plan is for two elders to take turns providing child care so that the other can participate in the group (Skalland, 1995).

When there is a case of domestic violence, even though screams may be heard, neighbors are afraid to call the police. Skalland and others formed a multidisciplinary elder abuse consultation team (MEACY), teaching, through ethnic media and foreign-language videos, that abuse is against the law here, that it must be reported, and how to report it.

A/PI communities require a broad range of services to meet existing needs. This not only involves creating culturally relevant and community-situated programs but also recruitment and training bilingual and bicultural A/PIs for direct service, community education, and prevention programs.

Ethnogerocounseling Terminations

A/PI clients who want to be courteous may find unique ways to terminate counseling. No-show clients may be dissatisfied with your service or may simply be uncertain about how and when to say good-bye. Koreans, who typically stress loyalty in relationships, may be overly sensitive if you suggest termination. So determine early on how each client has learned to handle separation and its effects, and also let the client know what to expect.

Another way a relationship terminates is, of course, through death. Chapter 14 covered some aspects of A/PIs' mores regarding death and dying. Just as members of a family or a group differ in beliefs and practices related to bereavement, ethnic groups differ too. Probably at no other time is it as important for you, the ethnogerocounselor, to be culturally aware and to act correctly. Thus you must learn about the prescribed death rituals of your client's ethnic family and group.

For the Japanese, there are necessary ceremonies performed by close family members at the time of death for the well-being of the soul. These include bathing and anointing the body and dressing it in a white kimono before it is removed by the eldest son or a priest. Family and friends visit with the deceased for two days, offering prayers, gifts, and money and burn incense. Americanization has shortened this complex process and cremation is often chosen, but afterward special ceremonial days (the seventh, forty-ninth, and hundredth day after the funeral) are observed.

Filipino men wear a black armband or a small black ribbon pinned to a shirt pocket, and women wear a black dress for a prescribed period of mourning, depending on the closeness of the relationship. A wreath draped in black adorns the family's door. Long obituaries appear in the newspapers, requesting prayers for the soul of the deceased and inviting friends to the funeral.

In contrast, Vietnamese Buddhists—who believe that karma determines death and rebirth—seldom share grief outside the intimate family. After death, the body is dressed in the deceased person's best clothes, a few grains of rice are placed in the mouth, and money is put in a pocket to pay for drinks. Friends who have been invited to call are announced to the deceased with music at each entrance. All wear white. Before the funeral procession and cremation, the family offers prayerful good-byes. Mourning continues for 100 days (AARP, 1990a).

Buddhists, who stress impermanence and reincarnation, believe that greed and hate produce suffering and repeated births in an unsatisfactory world; but a calm mind and compassionate behavior bring people closer to buddhahood.

Proper care of the body immediately after death influences the process of rebirth. Instructions are read to the dying person to help guide the consciousness through the transition (*bardo*) to the next life form; therefore, any psychoactive drugs (such as morphine) may be refused. A death that was violent, unexpected, or out of generational order is of concern, because it may agitate or disturb the mind.

Buddhists have no special burial rituals; cremation is often for people of status; children, holy men, and the poor are buried. While death is considered positive—an opportunity for improvement in the next life—family loyalty and custom allow for a show of grief such as wearing white headbands and armbands. Family members use walking sticks to symbolize their need for support. One comforts the bereaved by speaking of the deceased's good humor and clear mind at death (Wellen, 1995).

Among the Hmong, traditional beliefs about death center on animism, the soul, and the "house of three spirits." The Hmong believe that the physical and spiritual worlds coexist and that all of nature is inhabited by spirits. The duration of one's life depends on how one pleases the chief of the gods; but even though the date of death is predestined, discussion of death is forbidden in the presence of the dying, as that may hasten it. The spirit is believed to be lost and homeless if death takes place in a hospital, so it is better to die at home.

A body must be kept whole with no invasive procedures such as autopsy or organ donation. It is positioned so that the feet point toward an open window, so that the dead person will face a mountain or open space. All family work ceases until the burial; and for 13 days after death the departed soul is invited to share meals with the family (Wellen, 1995). Gold and silver paper is burned to symbolize the provision of money for the next life. The family's future health and safety depend on a proper burial. The older the deceased, the longer and more elaborate the funeral.

Yang (personal communication, 1997) said soon after receiving notice of a death, a counselor can call on the grieving person; but he or she should not ask for details about the death. It is okay to telephone for information about the funeral and to ask, "What can I do?" Flowers and money are appropriate gifts, but food is never given. At the funeral home, the recipient may bow many times until the donor acknowledges the thanks.

Yang said it is important to be aware that many Hmong have converted to Christianity and follow Christian practices.

Samoans—Polynesian natives of Guam, Hawaii, and American Samoa—like other ethnic groups, range from people who are highly acculturated to people, including many elders, who remain true to traditional ways. Many come to the mainland to visit for as long as a year or more or come to help out at times of illness and death. Most combine Christian and traditional Samoan beliefs and practices regarding religion and health.

Few elders use western medicine, often because of language problems. When they do, compliance and follow-up may falter. Usually the sick are cared for at home in consultation with their own elder healers (who use herbal remedies and teas). Many designated family caregivers who are already poor make great financial and personal sacrifices to care for a patient. Often, the family chips in to pay for a caregiver's airfare to the mainland. A bed may be purchased for a patient, but often the customary floor mat is preferred. When a person is hospitalized, the family stays at the hospital around the clock, on a rotating schedule; female family members feed, clean, and entertain the patient.

Among Samoans in the United States, a body is taken to a funeral home, where female relatives dress and place a lei on it for the viewing. Christian services are held at the funeral home and at the grave after the *matai* (family chief) has called all the relatives who are expected to attend. Then money ($1000 to $2000) is collected according to a complex method. Each relative is expected to contribute—the closer the relationship, the bigger the contribution—so that the family can pay in cash immediately at the end of the service.

If the bones of the deceased (particularly a *matai* or someone from a prominent family) are not treated respectfully, the spirit could cause trouble later: sickness, accidents, pain, death. Funeral directors know that they must provide a room holding at least 200 people for several days before the burial. This is for the services, and it needs to accommodate a large group of Samoan choir women, singers, and mourners who sit at the side of the coffin. Children are usually present. Sometimes *Aloha Oe* ("Love and farewell") or *Tofa, Tofa, Tofa* ("Farewell, Farewell, Good-bye") is sung.

Giving fine 4-foot by 5-foot pandanus mats is another important funeral ritual. Rare and no longer made, they cannot be taken out of American Samoa, so the custom is difficult to observe in the United States. A system of returns has been developed: purchased or loaned mats are returned to donors after the funeral.

Samoans view death as God's will, a natural event in life, and the family easily accepts replacement roles. "The coming together of the Samoan community at the time of death fosters a sense of caring and community which serves the family and friends well in their home away from Samoa" (King, 1990).

As with other ethnic groups and the dominant culture, such are the losses and discoveries, the sadness and joys, experienced in gerocounseling.

EXERCISE

Think again about the Asian/Pacific Island American elders who are described at the beginning of this part. On the basis of some of the principles of ethnogerocounseling discussed here, how would you devise a care or treatment plan for each person? How would your work differ from your work with elders and their families of the dominant culture? What more do you need to know? Include both micro and macro interventions.

References

American Association of Retired Persons. (1990a). *Customs of bereavement: A guide for providing cross-cultural assistance.* Washington, DC: AARP.

American Association of Retired Persons. (1990b). *Health risks and preventive care among older Pacific/Asian Americans.* Washington, DC: AARP.

American Association of Retired Persons. (1995). *A portrait of older minorities.* Washington, DC: AARP.

American Association of Retired Persons. (1996). *Appreciating diversity: A tool for building bridges.* Washington, DC: Author.

Browne, C., & Broderick, A. (1995). Asian and Pacific Island elders: Issues for social work practice and education. *Social Work, 40* (2), 252–259.

Burlingame, V. (1992). Report on travel to china with American Society on Aging. (Unpublished).

Hasegawa, K. (1989, March). Research update of cross-cultural aspects of Alzheimer's disease in Japan. Paper presented at the Asian-Pacific Alzheimer's Disease Conference, Honolulu, HI.

Ishisaka, H., & Takagi, C. (1982). Social work with Asian and Pacific-Americans. In J. W. Green (Ed.), *Cultural awareness in the human services.* Englewood Cliffs, NJ: Prentice Hall.

Kaneshige, E. (1973). Cultural factors in group counseling and interaction. *Personnel and Guidance Journal, 51,* 407–412.

Kii, T. (1984). Asians. In E. Palmore (Ed.), *Handbook on the aged in the United States.* Westport, CN: Greenwood.

Kim, P. (1990). Asian American families and the elderly. In U.S. Department of Health and Human Services, *Minority Aging.* Washington, DC: U.S. Public Health Service.

King, A. (1990). A Samoan perspective: Funeral practices, death, and dying. In J. Parry (Ed.), *Social work practice with the terminally ill: A transcultural perspective.* Springfield, IL: Thomas.

Kitano, H., & Daniels, R. (1988). *Asian Americans: Emerging minorities.* Englewood Cliffs, NJ: Prentice Hall.

Lee, J., Patchner, M., & Balgopal, P. (1991). Essential dimensions for developing and delivering service for the Asian American elderly. *Journal of Multicultural Social Work, 1,* 3–11.

Lieber, M. (1990). Lamarckian definitions of identity on Kapingamarangi and Pohnpei. In J. Linnekin & l. Poyer (Eds.), *Cultural identity and ethnicity in the Pacific.* Honolulu: University of Hawaii Press, pp. 1–15.

Lin, Tsung-Yi. (1983). Psychiatry and Chinese culture. In Cross-cultural medicine. *Western Journal of Medicine, 139,* 862–867.

Liu, W., & Yu, E. (1985). Asian/Pacific American elderly: Mortality differentials, health status, and use of health services. *Journal of Applied Gerontology, 4,* 35–64.

Locke, D. (1992). *Increasing multicultural understanding, A comprehensive model.* Newbury Park, CA: Sage.

Lum, O. (1993). *Chinese American elders.* Presentation on historical profiles of African-American, Latino, Filipino, and Chinese elders. Working Paper No. 12. Palo Alto, CA: Stanford Geriatric Education Center, 43–50.

McInnis, K., Petracchi, H., & Morgenbesser, M. (1990). *The Hmong in America: Providing ethnic-sensitive health, education, and human services.* Dubuque, IA: Kendall/Hunt.

Moroka-Douglas, N., & Yeo, G. (1990). *Aging and health: Asian/ Pacific Island American elders.* Stanford Geriatric Education Center Working Paper No. 3. Stanford, CA: SGEC.

Nakasone, R. (1990). *Ethics of enlightenment.* Fremont, CA: Dharma Cloud.

Nguyen, D. 91989). Discussion recorded at conference on *Traditional and Nontraditional Medication Use Among Ethnic Elders.* Stanford Geriatric Education Center Working Paper No. 10. Palo Alto, CA: SGEC.

Powell, G. (Ed.). (1983). *The psychosocial development of minority group children.* New York: Brunner/Mazel.

Sue, D.W., & Sue, D. (1990). *Counseling the culturally different: Theory and practice.* New York: Wiley.

Tien, J. (1984). Do Asians need less medication? *Journal of Psychosocial Nursing, 22,* 19–22.

Tseng, W., McDermott, J., & Maretzski, T. (Eds.) (1974). *The Chinese of Hawaii: People and cultures in Hawaii.* Honolulu: University of Hawaii School of Medicine.

Tsui, P., & Schultz, G. (1988). Ethnic factors in group process: Cultural dynamics in multi-ethnic therapy groups. *American Journal of Psychotherapy, 58,* 136–142.

U.S. Bureau of the Census. (1992). *1900 census of the population. General population characteristics. CP-1.* Washington, DC: Author.

U.S. Bureau of the Census and National Institute on Aging. (1993). Racial and ethnic diversity of America's elderly population. *Profiles of America's elderly, 3.* Washington, DC: Author.

Wellen, D. (1995, March 31). Cultural diversity and end of life issues: Death rituals and care of the body. Paper presented at the Cultural Diversity and End of Life Issues Conference, Stanford, CA: SGEC.

Yamamoto, J., & Iga, M. (1983). Emotional growth of Japanese children. In G. Powell (Ed.), *The psychosocial development of minority group children*. New York: Brunner/Mazel.

Yeo, G., & Hikoyeda, N. (1992). *Cohort analysis as a clinical and educational tool in ethnogeriatrics: Historical profiles of Chinese, Filipino, Mexican, and African American elders*. SGEC Working Paper. Palo Alto, CA: Stanford Geriatric Education Center.

Yeo, G. (1995, January). Ethical considerations in Asian/Pacific elders. *Clinics in Geriatric Medicine*.

Yeo, G., & Gallagher-Thompson, D. (Eds.). (1996). *Ethnicity and the Dementias*. Washington, DC: Taylor and Francis.

Yesavage, J., Brink, T., Rose, T., Lum, O., Huang, V., Adey, M., & Leirer, V. (1983). Development and validation of a geriatric depression screening scale: A preliminary report. *Journal of Psychiatric Research 17*, 37–49.

Yu, K., & Kim, L. (1983). The growth and development of Korean-American children. In G. Powell (Ed.), *The psychosocial development of minority group children*. New York: Brunner/Mazel.

Acknowledgements for Part V

I thank the Geriatric Education Center at Stanford University, Palo Alto, California for generously sharing hard-to-find current literature on ethnicity, aging, and Asian/Pacific Island American elders. Many individuals also helped in the preparation of this chapter.

I wish to also thank the A/PI health and social service providers and experts who either took time out of their busy schedules to grant me interviews or presented materials at workshops that I attended.

From San Jose, California: Owen Lum, MD, at Santa Teresa Kaiser Medical Center; Shari Skalland, MSW, Gerontology Supervisor at the Cypress Senior Center; and Carlina Yeung, MSW, and Hsiu-Lan Lu, MSW, Counselors at Asian Americans for Community Involvement. In San Mateo: Karen Lam, MSW, Center Director and Francis Huang, MSW, Counselor, at Self Help for the Elderly, San Mateo Center; and Roz Enomoto at the San Mateo Japanese American Citizens League. Others who helped were: Doreen McLeod,

MSW, Director at On Lok in San Francisco; Linda S. Wahl, MA, Administrator, and Calvin M. Hara, MA, Assistant Administrator, at the Asian Community Nursing Home in Sacramento; Melen McBride, RN, PhD at Stanford Geriatric Education Center; and Alice Bulos, PhD, activist, in South San Francisco.

I also thank Lee Hovag-Spitz, MA, gerontologist, in Boston; and Miva Yang, RN, at the Sheboygan, Wisconsin, County Health Department.

Epilogue

Throughout the 1990s, a task force from the Office of Management and Budget and the U.S. Census spent over $5 million consulting hundreds of experts on an awkward question: What kind of American are you in terms of a basic racial and ethnic category? It is an important question because not only are federal policies, programs, and research involved, but an accurate picture of the United States is at stake. Many people abhor ethnic labels because they tend to perpetuate attention to racial differences and because like Bessie Delaney, they just want to be called Americans. But others argue that ethnic labels also ensure a certain protection, aid, and a check on inequities.

Despite a growing preference for a multiracial category, the current task force rejected it as too confusing. The new changes agreed upon as of this writing will be as follows: Black should become Black or African American with Haitian or Negro also allowed. Hispanic will be kept, but Latino or Spanish Origin will be permitted. American Indian will be retained. Hawaiian will become Native Hawaiian. Not everyone is pleased.

Another important issue has to do with the ambivalence in the dominant society—and even among ethnic peoples—about whether everyone should be treated the same or, out of sensitivity, pragmatism, or respect for the differences of others, we should tailor our behaviors to meet the unique needs and circumstances of ethnic peoples in culturally sensitive, culturally competent ways. This too is not an easy problem to solve. There are some who want it answered just one way, some who seem to want it answered both ways, and some who are looking for a workable compromise.

Many people believe that the dream of a melting pot did not materialize because the message of the dominant society to immigrants seemed to be, "Now *you* can become just like *us*." Except for sampling ethnic foods, looking in on ethnic festivals, attending powwows on a vacation, posting bilingual signs in airports, or applauding black athletes or entertainers, the dominant culture seldom suggested that its members might become more like "ethnics." As with our policies for American Indians, the plan was to ultimately erase alien cultures, not to absorb or incorporate them. No wonder that immigrating societies hung on tenaciously to their ethnic roots. This was not just due to pride or to a need for security; erasure would mean giving up much of value.

This is especially evident with regard to aging. As the United States enters a new millennium, it faces the problem of an increasing elderly population concurrent with shrinking resources. And since we are told that the government can no longer "do it all," the dominant society might well look to its ethnic kin for guidance.

Eighteenth- and nineteenth-century American values of independence and self-sufficiency may have to give way to ethnic ideas of interdependence, reciprocity between generations, and a flexible family-centered (not self-centered) basic unit. Buddhist ideas about impermanence would be of help to elders struggling with losses; the black culture's incredible support system and the survival skills of its elder members could be adopted into our repertoires of coping; and already many elders are looking to ethnic cures to meet some problems of aging less expensively and less invasively.

A model of older persons is like a model of all age groups in terms of basic needs and wants, but we must also add a Gero Chi Lens to include unique tasks and circumstances of aging. This will enable us to be more sensitive and more competent as regards aging persona. But of course we must understand that there is more variability within the older population than within any other age group.

Likewise, even though ethnic older persons are like all other older persons in terms of basic needs, wants, and tasks, we must apply an Ethnic Lens to the Gero Chi Lens so that we can be more ethnic sensitive and more competent with regard to ethnicity. But here too we must understand that there is much variability among ethnic groups. This will cause us to rethink many of our old ways of viewing and offering services to ethnic elders and their families.

Maybe we will even have to rethink the golden rule! Instead of "treat others as you would like to be treated," the rule could be rephrased: "Treat others as they would like to be treated." Such is the thesis of this book.

Index

Springer Publishing Company

Aging in Rural Settings
Life Circumstances and Distinctive Features of Aging in Rural America

Raymond T. Coward, MSW, PhD
John A. Krout, PhD, Editors

This text offers readers a concise state of the art summary of the critical dimensions of growing old in rural environments. Prominent researchers explore topical areas that focus on life conditions, diversity, services, and public policies for rural elders. For students, this book provides a comprehensive overview of the field, addressing challenges that dominate this field of study. For experienced ruralists, this book is a useful reference tool that brings together in one place the writings of a diverse, wide-spread, and constantly growing body of literature.

Contents:

1998   320pp   0-8261-9720-5   *hardcover*

536 Broadway, New York, NY 10012-3955 • (212) 431-4370 • Fax (212) 941-7842

⑤ *Springer Publishing Company*

Religion, Belief, and Spirituality in Late Life

L. Eugene Thomas, PhD, Susan A. Eisenhandler, PhD

This volume examines the importance of beliefs in understanding psychologically-relevant issues from self-identity to recovery from grief. Thomas and Eisenhandler provide a broad framework for viewing religion in the lives of the elderly by drawing on insights derived from the humanities, and those mined from qualitative social science research, as well as from empirical and quantitative research.

This book is a valuable resource for academics, gerontologists, psychologists, graduate-level students, and other professionals who are interested in the emerging study of religion, spirituality, and aging.

1998   248pp (est.)   0-8261-1235-8   hardcover

536 Broadway, New York, NY 10012-3955 • (212) 431-4370 • Fax (212) 941-7842

SP *Springer Publishing Company*

Gerontological Social Work
Theory Into Practice

Ilene L. Nathanson, DSW, BCD
Terry T. Tirrito, DSW

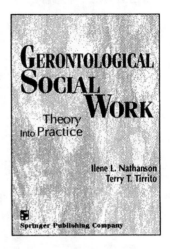

In this book, the authors develop a conceptual framework for task-centered social work practice with older adults. Their integrative model clearly illustrates how practitioners and students should incorporate social work practices in various settings including psychiatric, health, religious, legal, occupational, and more. Material on communication skills makes the volume more useful for students learning to work with the elderly. The authors' stimulating case studies make this an ideal text for undergraduate and graduate social work programs in gerontology.

Contents:

- Social Work Practice Revisited
- Integrative Model of Gerontological Social Work
- Specialized Needs of Older People
- Gerontological Psychiatric Social Work Practice
- Social Work With the Aging in a Legal Environment
- Gerontological Social Work Practice and the Religious
  Environment
- Communication Skills for Gerontological Social Work Practice
- The Integrative Model of Gerontological Social Work

1997   176pp   0-8261-9890-2   hardcover

536 Broadway, New York, NY 10012-3955 • (212) 431-4370 • Fax (212) 941-7842

SP *Springer Publishing Company*

Multicultural Perspectives in Working with Families

Elaine P. Congress, DSW

"Elaine Congress's new book is an extremely useful text, on the cutting edge of this emerging and critical issue for our field and our world. The book is well-written, thoughtful, and full of practical insights to help therapists develop their work in this area."

—**Monica McGoldrick,** PhD
Director, Family Institute of New Jersey

"This excellent volume brings wisdom to all who wish to become truly multicultural practitioners—wisdom that is practical, complex, and useful. The author avoids focus on specific characteristics of different populations and shows the reader how to learn about and understand the experiences, the values, the meanings of people who live in different worlds and to translate that understanding into helpful practice."

—**Ann Hartman,** DSW
Dean Emerita, Smith College, School for Social Work

"It is a 'must read' for beginning and advanced practitioners."

—**Jesse J. Harris,** DSW
Dean and Professor, University of Maryland,
School of Social Work

Written for social work practitioners, educators, and students, this important volume seeks to deflate stereotypes and promote unbiased thinking. Carrying forward the updated curriculum policy on cultural diversity of the Council on Social Work Education, the key topics addressed include HIV/AIDS, homelessness, substance abuse, domestic violence, and child sexual abuse.

Contents:
- Assessment—Micro and Macro Approaches
- Culturally Diverse Families Across the Life Cycle
- Selected Culturally Diverse Populations
- Challenging Practice Issues
- Beyond Family Therapy

Springer Series on Social Work
1997   376pp   0-8261-9560-1   *hardcover*

536 Broadway, New York, NY 10012-3955 • (212) 431-4370 • Fax (212) 941-7842